Teaching the Medical/Surgical Patient
Diagnostics and Procedures

Triphy C. Barber, RN, MT, PhD
Dot E. Langfitt, RN, BA, MN, CCRN

Robert J. Brady Co.
A Prentice-Hall Publishing and Communications Company
Bowie, MD 20715

Executive Editor: Richard Weimer
Production Editor/Text Design: Paula Huber
Art Director: Don Sellers, AMI
Assistant Art Director: Bernard Vervin

Indexer: Nancy Bailey
Typesetter: Harper Graphics, Waldorf, MD
Printer: Port City Press, Baltimore, MD
Typeface: Univers

Teaching the Medical/Surgical Patient: Diagnostics and Procedures

Library of Congress Cataloging in Publication Data

Barber, Triphy C., 1946—
  Teaching the medical/surgical patient.

  1. Diagnosis. 2. Patient education. 3. Nursing.
I. Langfitt, Dot E., 1941— . II. Title. [DNLM:
1. Diagnostic tests, Routine—Nursing texts. 2. Patient
education—Nursing texts. WY 105 B234t]
RT48.B37 1983   616.07′5   83-2533
ISBN 0-89303-881-4

Prentice-Hall International, Inc., London
Prentice-Hall Canada, Inc., Scarborough, Ontario
Prentice-Hall of Australia, Pty., Ltd., Sydney
Prentice-Hall of India Private Limited, New Delhi
Prentice-Hall of Japan, Inc., Tokyo
Prentice-Hall of Southeast Asia Pte. Ltd., Singapore
Whitehall Books, Limited, Petone, New Zealand
Editora Prentice-Hall Do Brasil LTDA., Rio de Janeiro

Printed in the United States of America

83 84 85 86 87 88 89 90 91 92 93 10 9 8 7 6 5 4 3 2 1

Contents

Preface

At the beginning of each group of diagnostic procedures, there is a section for the nurse. The information in this section briefly defines the procedure, explains its indications, how it is done, and what the responsibilities are for pre- and post-care of the patient undergoing the procedure.

Directly following the Nurse's Guide are individual Patient Guides to the specific procedures ordered by the physician. **These Patient Guides are to be photocopied and given to the patients (and family) for their information.** At the end of each Patient Guide is a place for the patients or members of their family to write comments or questions.

It is our hope that the Nurse's and Patient Guides to the specific diagnostic procedures discussed in this book will lead to better understanding by patients and their family. We also hope that this book will help to further the quality and continuity of care by the health staff.

Triphy C. Barber
Dot E. Langfitt

This book is dedicated, with love,
To my husband, Clifford,
for his support and understanding

To my parents, Elaine and John,
in appreciation of their support and encouragement

TB

To my mother and father,
and all other patients
who will benefit from clear explanations of their test procedures

DL

1
Radiographic Procedures

Diagnostic Ultrasound

This procedure may be called ultrasonography or sonography. It is a noninvasive procedure and is used to study the internal structures of the body in a two- or three-dimensional plane.

Ultrasound is done by measuring the time interval of the transmission of ultrasonic waves to the reflections of the sound waves off tissue, liquid, or bone. This procedure is done with the aid of a transducer and an ultrasonic machine. This machine contains an oscilloscope for visualization of the structure being studied. The information is stored by photographic film or other means for study by a radiologist.

This procedure may be used to study multiple areas, which include brain (mid-line), heart and great vessels, lymph nodes, stomach, gallbladder, spleen, liver, pancreas, kidneys, ureters, and fetus.

Nurse's Responsibilities

Pre-Test
1. Explain procedure to patient and family.
2. Assist in getting patient ready for transport or, if done at bedside, help position patient.
3. Have patient void before procedure.

Precautions
None.

Post-Procedure Care
1. Make patient comfortable.
2. Help patient to remove any ultrasonic gel that may not have been removed post procedure.

Nuclear Studies

Nuclear studies use the aid of radioisotopes to study the internal physiologic processes of the body. This is done by measuring the amount of emitted radiation from an injected radioisotope.

These tests are an invasive study due to the fact that a radioisotope is injected directly into the venous system.

Below is a brief description of the body systems that may be studied and the purposes for doing the studies.

1. *BRAIN SCAN*—Normally a radioisotope cannot penetrate the blood-brain barrier. However, in pathological states where the barrier has been broken down, the radioisotope will show the abnormality.

Purpose of Study:
a. To identify intracranial tumors or other vascular lesions.
b. To evaluate the course of post-surgical lesions and tumors.
c. To evaluate lesions during the course of chemo- and radiation therapy.
d. To locate intracranial bleeding (hemorrhage) and areas of ischemia or actual infarct.

2. *HEART SCAN*—There are three particular scans done in this group (thallium imaging, cardiac gated pool imaging, and technetium imaging). Of the three groups, thallium imaging is the most popular.

Purpose of Studies:
a. *Thallium Imaging:*
(1) To evaluate the patient with an acute or past myocardial infarction (M.I.)
(2) To assess myocardial scarring due to infarction or trauma.
(3) To assess myocardial perfusion and through stress exercise, to diagnose probable coronary artery disease.
(4) To evaluate post-surgical grafts and/or transluminal angioplasty.
(5) To evaluate drug therapy.
b. *Cardiac Gated Pool Imaging:*
(1) Most critical is the evaluation of left ventricular function.
(2) To demonstrate intracardiac shunting of blood.
(3) To evaluate myocardial wall motion function as a whole.
c. *Technetium Scanning:*
(1) Confirmation of a recent M.I.
(2) Evaluation of size, location, and prognosis post M.I.

3. *PULMONARY SCANS*—Pulmonary scans are divided into two groups (lung perfusion and lung ventilation). These tests are often done simultaneously, especially when looking for pulmonary emboli.

Purpose of Studies:
a. *Lung Perfusion Studies:*
(1) To demonstrate pulmonary emboli.
(2) To evaluate the patient with regional hypoventilation and respiratory function.

(3) To identify areas in the lung that may become (have the capacity) ventilated.

4. *ENDOCRINE STUDIES*—The most frequently studied organs in this category are the thyroid and pancreas. (The pancreas may also be listed under G.I. Studies.)

Purpose of Studies:
 a. *Thyroid:*
   (1) To assess thyroid function
   (2) To locate the thyroid and evaluate its size and structure.
   (3) To demonstrate any lesions.
 b. *Pancreas:*
   (1) To assess pancreatic function.
   (2) To locate the gland and evaluate its size and structure.
   (3) To demonstrate any lesions.

5. *GASTROINTESTINAL SYSTEM*—The liver and spleen are usually studied together in this system. However, the spleen may also be studied in hemopoietic blood system.

Purpose of Study:
 a. To detect enlargement of the liver and spleen.
 b. To detect tumors, cysts, or other lesions of the liver and spleen.
 c. To evaluate the liver for hepatitis, cirrhosis, or other disease entities.
 d. To evaluate the liver and spleen post trauma.

6. *RENAL SCANS*—These studies may be done on persons who are allergic to contrast media.

Purpose of Study:
 a. To assess renal function.
 b. To detect renal obstruction.
 c. To assess renal structure and structure abnormalities.
 d. To evaluate the renal system post-trauma.
 e. To detect tumors or other focal lesions of the renal system.

7. *OTHER STUDIES*—There are many other scans that may be done (eye, bone, placental, hemopoietic, etc.). The purpose of these studies is much the same as listed above. To name but a few purposes, they include to evaluate function, to detect lesions, and to assess structure.

Nurse's Responsibilities

Pre-Test
 1. Explain procedure to patient and family.
 2. Explain that the isotopes will not cause radiation damage to the patient or family members.
 3. Ask the patient if he or she is allergic to fish or contrast media.
 4. Have patient void before taking patient to Nuclear Medicine. Average length of test is from one to two hours.
 5. Have patient ready for transport with chart to Nuclear Medicine.
 6. In a few of the nuclear procedures, the radioisotopes are given 1-2 hours prior to the procedure.

Precautions
 1. In the lung perfusion test, allergy to contrast media is contraindicated.
 2. Patient should be cooperative.

Post-Procedure Care
 1. Make patient comfortable.
 2. Resume prior orders.
 3. If hematoma is present at injection site, a warm compress may alleviate discomfort.

Computerized Axial Tomography Scanning (CT Scan or CAT Scan)

A CAT scan is a dual radiographic unit comprised of a computer and radiographic scanner. The radiographic scanner produces a fan-like beam of radiation through a section of tissue being studied. Multiple radiation detectors then measure the intensity of this beam after it has passed through the section. The computer, through complex mathematical formulae, calculates the amount of radiation absorbed by the body section. The computer reconstructs an image or picture of that section.

CAT scans are done for numerous reasons. The most common are to aid in the diagnosis of tumors and lesions and to follow their course post-chemo and/or radiotherapy.

Other Differences Between Conventional X-Ray Machine and CAT Scan

A regular x-ray machine emits a focused beam of radiation through a section of the body. The organs or tissue closest to the x-ray source are superimposed over the organs furthest from the x-ray. This results in a two-dimensional (flat) picture of a three-dimensional organ. This information is then stored on photographic film.

The CAT Scanner, like the conventional x-ray unit, also produces a two-dimensional picture. However, here the similarity ends. Due to the numerous cross-sectional views or slices that are projected on the television-like screen, the radiologist is able to obtain the depth effect, thus giving the organ a three-dimensional view.

CAT Scans, due to their use of radiation and contrast media for tissue enhancement, are considered to be an invasive procedure.

Nurse's Responsibilities

Pre-Test
 1. Explain procedure to patient and family.
 2. This procedure may be done on an out-patient basis.
 3. Patient should be asked to get into a hospital gown and to void prior to the scan.
 4. If contrast media is to be used, ask the patient if he or she is allergic to shellfish or iodine products.
 5. Patient may be NPO for procedure if contrast media is used. Normally, NPO post midnight

unless procedure is scheduled in the P.M. If this is the case, light (clear liquid) breakfast may be given.
6. Make sure patient and chart are ready for transport to the radiographic department.

Precautions
1. The contrast media used for enhancement is usually an iodine base dye. If the patient is allergic to shellfish or dye, the physician needs to be notified. This is a contraindication for this part of the procedure. (Some physicians may elect to continue with the procedure after the patient has been prepped with steroids.)
2. Food and fluids are withheld prior to the test if contrast media is used due to a chance of nausea or vomiting occurring upon intravenous injection of the dye.
3. The CAT Scan procedure room should contain emergency equipment and medications.

Post-Procedure Care
1. Make patient as comfortable as possible.
2. Resume pre-procedure orders.
3. If hematoma is present at injection site, a warm compress may ease the discomfort.
4. If contrast media was used, encourage an increased oral intake and note time and amount of patient's first voiding.

Angiography

An angiographic procedure is the study of one or more blood vessels in the body. This procedure is usually broken down into two distinct categories: arteriograms (study of the arteries) and venograms (study of the veins). Together or separately, these studies are called angiograms.

Any organ or area that has a blood supply may be studied by angiography. When a particular area of study has been chosen by the radiologist, the study is called selective angiography of the particular tissue. (For example, selective study of the carotid arteries.)

Angiography is an invasive procedure less used in primary diagnosis due to the advent of less invasive procedures (nuclear medicine, ultrasound, and CAT scan). It is still, however, of great benefit in conformation of the extent of tumors and lesions, and in the diagnosis of abnormalities of the vascular system (stenosis, aneurysms, blockage, and hemorrhage).

Nurse's Responsibilities

Pre-Test
1. Explain the procedure to the patient and family. Explain that when the dye is injected, he or she will feel a very warm sensation and some discomfort. This feeling will only last a few seconds and it is very important that he or she does not move.

2. Obtain a written permit for the procedure.
3. Patient will be NPO post-midnight for the test.
4. Ask the patient and check the chart for any allergies to shellfish or iodine products.
5. Help the patient into a hospital gown and ask him or her to void.
6. Premedicate the patient as per orders.
7. If patient does not have an IV going, call for an order and start an IV with an 18g or larger needle.
8. Have patient and chart ready for transfer to the radiographic suite.

Precautions
1. Patient should be cooperative. If not, call radiology to let them know the patient is restless.
2. Allergy to contrast media (iodine base) is contraindicated for the procedure unless the physician first preps the patient with steroids.
3. Contrast media may cause nausea and/or vomiting. Thus, the patient is kept NPO prior to the procedure.
4. Contrast media is excreted via the kidneys; thus, a recent BUN should be in the chart for the physician.
5. The special procedure area should contain emergency equipment and medications.

Post-Procedure Care
1. Make patient as comfortable as possible.
2. Check vital signs as per order (q15 min X4, q30 min X4, q1 hr X4 and q4 hr).
3. Check catheter insertion site for drainage, bleeding, redness, or signs of hematoma.
4. Instruct the patient to stay in bed 4 to 8 hours or as per order.
5. Encourage fluids.
6. Note time and amount of first voiding.
7. Give analgesics and sedatives as per order.
8. Check chart for orders pertinent for specific angiograms.

Radiation Therapy

Radiation therapy is one mode of treating carcinoma. It may be used alone or in combination with chemotherapy or surgery.

Radiation therapy utilizes x-ray, cobalt, linear accelerators, implants, and other sources of radiation to treat disease.

Nurse's Responsibilities

Pre-Test
1. Explain procedure to patient and family. This will have been done by the physician and/or radiologist but often the patient and family need reinforcement. Explain that procedure is often done on an out-patient basis.
2. Obtain a written permit. Again, this is often done by the physician.

3. Have patient put on a gown and void.
4. This procedure is often done as an out-patient.

Precautions
1. Prior to the first procedure, the patient often goes to the radiation therapy department for an evaluation and further studies. The radiologist may draw on the patient's skin where it will be irradiated. Tell the patient not to wash these marks off.
2. The patient should protect this area from sunlight (further radiation) and other things which may cause tissue damage.
3. It is important that the patient eat as normally as possible and receive enough sleep.
4. Stress that it is important during this time that the patient does not practice "self-treatment" for minor aches or pains. The physician should be contacted before any medication or treatment is done.
5. If a radioactive implant is used, the patient should be isolated and traffic in and out of the room be kept to a minimum.

Post-Procedure Care
1. Make patient as comfortable as possible.
2. Encourage the patient to keep as normal a life style as possible during treatments.
3. Examine marked area to ensure that the tissue integrity has not been broken.

NOTE: Pregnant nurses should not be exposed to radiation of any type.

Your Guide to Diagnostic Ultrasound

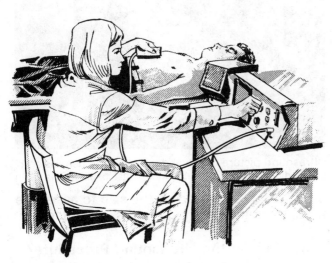

Patient being scanned with ultrasound.

What Is Diagnostic Ultrasound?

Diagnostic ultrasound is sometimes referred to as **ultrasonography** or **sonography**. It is used in studying internal structures of the body. It works in a similar manner to sonar on a submarine that finds other ships.

Why Is the Procedure Done?

Diagnostic ultrasound is done to visualize internal structures and soft tissues of the body to aid in the diagnosis of disease. This technique allows the physician to study areas of the body that previously could not be studied without using a surgical procedure.

What Organs Can Be Imaged With Ultrasound?

The ultrasound procedure may be done on a single part of the body, such as the kidneys, or on multiple parts of the body. These areas may include the spleen, liver, stomach, gallbladder, kidneys, pancreas, brain, lymph nodes, heart and great vessels, and fetus.

How Is the Procedure Done?

In ultrasonography, very high sound waves or **frequencies** (much higher than we can hear) are directed by a transducer toward the organ to be studied. A **transducer** is an electro-me-chanical device that can change one form of energy into another. In ultrasound, electrical energy is converted into sound waves. The sound waves that come in contact with internal structures in the body are reflected back to the skin surface where they are picked up by the transducer. In turn, these ultrasonic waves are electronically converted to visual images (pictures) of the structure which is being studied. These pictures are displayed on a type of television screen called an **oscilloscope**. These pictures or images can then be photographed for storage and further study by a radiologist.

Where Is the Procedure Done?

Ultrasound is most often a part of the X-ray or radiology department. However, there are two special subdivisions known as echocardiography (ultrasound of the heart) and obstetric ultrasound (study of placenta and fetus). These may be done in other areas of the hospital. Some physicians may have ultrasound equipment in their office.

What Is Real-Time Ultrasound?

Through technological advances, a multi-channel transducer has been developed. Up to this time, ultrasound has been done with a single transducer. The use of the multi-channel

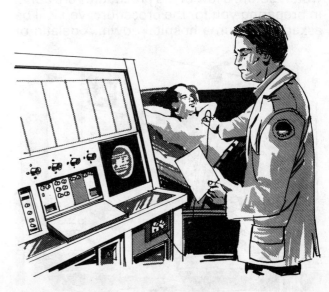

Studying internal organs with ultrasound.

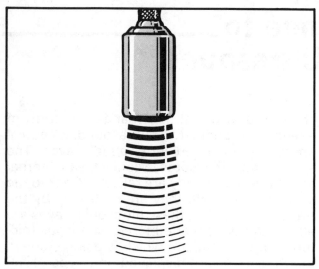
Transducer producing sound waves.

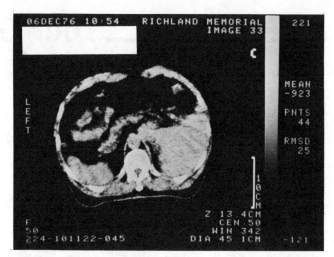
Ultrasound picture of the abdomen. (By permission of the Radiology Dept., Richland Memorial Hospital, Cola, SC.)

transducer allows the ultrasound technologist to observe and record movement of an organ within the body. These images or pictures are then recorded. They look similar to a motion picture. A most important principle in real-time ultrasound is that movement can be observed and recorded as it is actually occurring. This has been a major breakthrough in the field of cardiology. **Cardiology** is the study of the heart and great vessels.

Is There Any Preparation For This Procedure?

No! This procedure may be done on an in-patient or an out-patient basis. There are no time constraints on the time of the day or whether the patient has or has not eaten. There may be some special preparation, like drinking water, before a few of the procedures are done. In preparing you for the procedure, you will be asked to put on a hospital gown. A gelatin or oil will then be placed on the skin to assist the transducer in obtaining good skin contact.

Who Will Do the Ultrasound Procedure?

Today, due to the technological advances, ultrasound is run by a highly trained professional team. The ultrasound technologist will do the actual procedure, and then the data and pictures obtained from the procedure will be given to a radiologist. A **radiologist** is a physician who specializes in the use of radiation and radioactive materials for medical diagnosis and treatment.

How Long Does the Procedure Take?

This is a very difficult question to answer. The average time is about an hour. This may vary, depending upon the patient as well as the procedure.

Are There Any Complications Or Side Effects to the Ultrasound Procedure?

No! Ultrasound is painless. You will be aware of the ultrasound technologist moving the transducer across the skin surface but you will feel no discomfort.

Will the Ultrasound Procedure Be Covered By My Insurance?

Almost all insurance companies will pay the majority of the ultrasonic procedure costs. These costs will include the additional physician fee. The amount of the coverage will differ from one insurance company to another.

If you have any other questions, please contact your doctor.

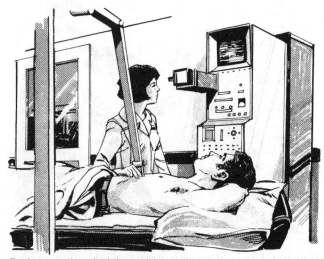
Patient and technician with oscilloscope.

Your Guide to Nuclear Studies

Introduction

Your doctor has requested that you have a special nuclear study done. It is important that you understand what this procedure is and why it is being done.

Terms pertaining to nuclear procedures, and the answers to some of the most frequently asked questions about nuclear studies, are contained in this guide.

What Is Nuclear Medicine?

Nuclear medicine is a branch of radiology that deals with the use of radioactive materials (radioisotopes) in medical diagnosis and treatment.

What Is Nuclear Study?

A **nuclear study** is the technique of studying normal functional processes of the body by measuring the amount of emitted radiation from a radioisotope.

What Area of the Body Can Be Studied with Nuclear Medicine?

- Brain (neurology studies)
- Heart (cardiovascular studies)
- Lungs (pulmonary studies)
- Bone (orthopedic studies)
- Pancreatic, Thyroid (endocrine studies)
- Kidneys (renal studies)
- Stomach, Liver (gastrointestinal studies)
- Blood Volume, Spleen (hemopoietic studies)
- Placental (genital studies)
- Eye Tumor (ophthalmology studies)
- Many Others

Why Is a Nuclear Study Done?

In simple terms, nuclear studies allow the physician to determine how an area of the body is functioning. These studies have replaced more involved, and invasive radiologic procedures.

Why a Nuclear Study Instead of a CT Scan or Ultrasound?

Ultrasound, computerized tomography scanning (CT scanning), and nuclear are all very useful diagnostic techniques that are mostly non-invasive in nature. (**Non-invasive** means not utilizing surgery, radiation, or intravenous/intra-arterial contrast media or dye.) Each of these diagnostic techniques measures a different physical variable or parameter. The recorded results of these techniques are an anatomic picture or representation of that physical variable.

Ultrasound measures the transmission of sound from an object (similar in principle to radar or sonar). CT scanning measures radiographic (X-ray) densities, or thickness of an object. A nuclear study measures a physiologic (functional) parameter.

What Is a Radioactive Isotope (Radioisotope)?

A **radioisotope** is an unstable isotope that decays to a stable state by emitting or giving off characteristic radiation.

How Is a Radioisotope Used?

A radioisotope is used in two different ways. The first manner in which it is used is for its radiation effect (diagnostic and therapeutic). The second manner in which it is used is as a tracer element added to a stable form

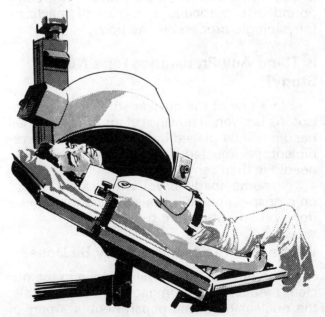

Patient in nuclear laboratory.

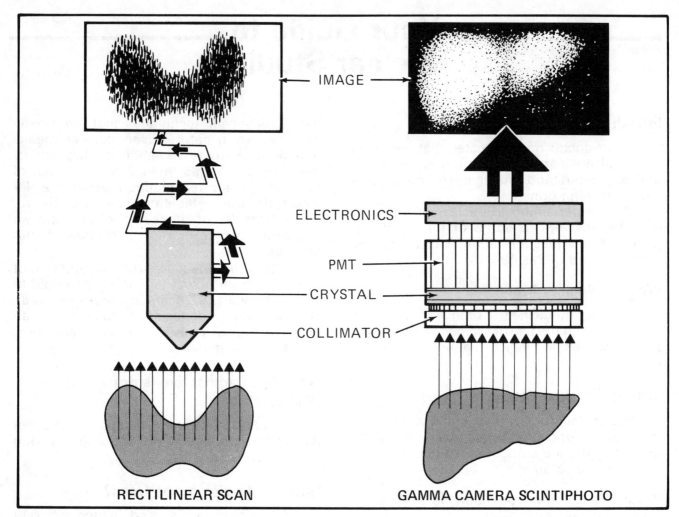

IMAGE

ELECTRONICS

PMT

CRYSTAL

COLLIMATOR

RECTILINEAR SCAN

GAMMA CAMERA SCINTIPHOTO

Diagram of cameras used for nuclear studies.

of a compound to follow the course of the compound in a particular sequence of reactions (physiologic process) in the body.

Is There Any Preparation for a Nuclear Study?

In a few of the nuclear studies, the radioisotope is given in advance of the study. A small needle will be placed in your vein, and the radioisotope injected through the needle. The needle is then removed.

In some hospitals you will be asked to put on a hospital gown, or this procedure may be done on an out-patient basis.

Where Will the Nuclear Study Be Done?

The nuclear study will be done in the nuclear medicine department. In most hospitals, the nuclear medicine department is a part of the radiology (X-ray) department.

Who Will Do the Study?

Nuclear studies, like many other procedures, utilize the team approach. The team members are highly trained nuclear technologists and a physician who specializes in radiation and radioactive materials used for medical diagnosis.

How Is the Nuclear Study Done?

You will be taken to the nuclear medicine department. There you will be helped onto a table, and made as comfortable as possible. If the radioisotope has not already been given, it will be at this time. A camera or scanner will be positioned over the area to be studied. The nuclear technologist may ask you to move from side to side, but other than positioning, you will lie still for most of the study. You will feel no discomfort. This is similar to having an X-ray or your picture taken.

In a few nuclear studies you will be asked to do specific functions. For example, in pulmonary perfusion studies you will be asked to breath into a bag. In the thallium exercise study, you will be asked to pedal a bicycle.

How Long Will the Nuclear Studies Take?

The time will vary with the type of study you are having done. Allow at least an hour to an hour and a half.

Does the Radioisotope Make Me Radioactive?

The answer to this question would have to be yes, but in a very limited manner. The radioisotope given to you for this procedure has a very short life span and *is not* very concentrated or strong.

How Long Will the Radioisotope Last in My Body?

This again will depend on what type of radioisotope was used. Most of the radioisotopes have short half lives, which means that the radiation level given off by the radioisotope drops very quickly.

Will the Radiation Hurt Me?

No! The dosages of the radioisotopes are carefully computed so that they will *not* be harmful to you!

When Will I Know the Results?

Your physician will discuss the results from the nuclear study with you and your family when they are received from the nuclear medicine department.

Are There Any Complications or Side Effects?

No!

Will My Insurance Cover This Procedure?

Most health insurance companies will cover the nuclear procedure as well as the physician fee. The amount of coverage will differ from one insurance company to another.

Comments and Questions

Terminology

Absorbed dose—the energy absorbed by the patient from the decay of the radioisotope.

Decay (radioactive)—the proportion of atoms of any radioactive substance that will disintegrate per unit of time.

Disintegration—the radioactive decay of one atom.

Half life—the time necessary for the concentration of the radioisotope to fall to one half its original concentration.

Isotope—an element with the same proton number (atomic) but different mass numbers (atomic weights C612 and C614).

Nuclear—pertaining to or constituting a nucleus.

Nuclear Medicine—the branch of medicine that deals with radioisotopes in diagnosis and therapy.

Nucleus—the core of an atom consisting of protons, neutrons, and alpha particles.

Radiation—the emission (giving off) of energy through space or through a material medium (solid, liquid) in a form having certain characteristic waves.

Radio—combining form—radiation, radium, radioactivity.

Radioactive—spontaneous decay of an unstable atomic nucleus.

Radioisotope—an unstable isotope that decays to a stable state by emitting characteristic radiation.

Radioisotope Camera (Scintillation)—one or more radiation counters that visualize a radioisotope deposition, with the camera in a fixed position in relation to the patient.

Radioisotope Scanner (Scintillation)—one or more radiation counters that visualize a radiosiotope deposition, with the scanner movable in relation to the patient.

Scintigram—a picture (image) of the distribution of radioactivity obtained with a radioisotope camera or scanner after the injection of a radioisotope.

Tracer—an isotope, that due to its unique physical properties, can be detected in small amounts, and used to trace a physiologic process by combining with a natural element.

Your Guide to
The CAT Scanner

What Is a CAT Scanner?

A **CAT scanner** (the abbreviated way of saying computerized axial tomography scanner) is a dual unit. It comprises a highly sophisticated computer and an X-ray machine. You also may have heard this machine referred to as a CT Scanner or computerized tomography scanner. For simplicity, we will refer to this machine as a CAT scanner.

What Is the Difference Between a "Head" and a "Whole-Body" Scanner?

The head scanner was the first machine developed. It could only do scans of the brain. As technology advanced, a whole body scanner was developed. This scanner can do brain scans and also various body scans.

How Does a CAT Scanner Work?

A CAT scanner produces a fan-like beam of radiation through a section of the body organ being studied. The computer calculates the amount of radiation absorbed by the body section. The computer then reconstructs an image or picture of that section. This information is stored on tape, disc, or photographic film.

Why Is a CAT Scan Done?

CAT scanners provide much better pictures of soft tissue than conventional X-rays.

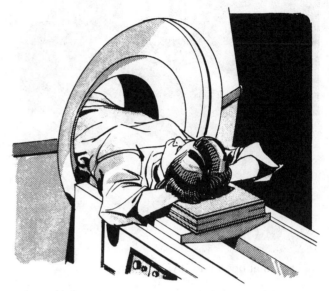
Whole body scanner.

A conventional X-ray picture will show only the differences in density (thickness) between air, bone, and soft tissue. The CAT scanner will show very fine density differences in the same tissue (normal tissue, blood, fluids, cancer, etc.).

Where Is a CAT Scan Done?

A CAT scan is done in a specialized area in the department of radiology in a hospital.

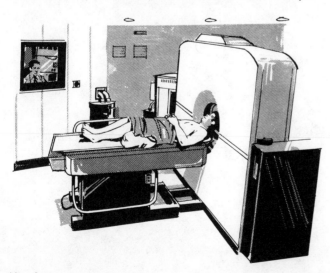
Head scanner.

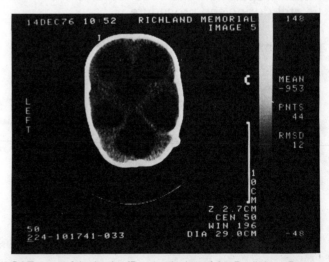
CAT scan of the brain. (By permission of the Radiology Dept., Richland Memorial Hospital, Cola, SC.)

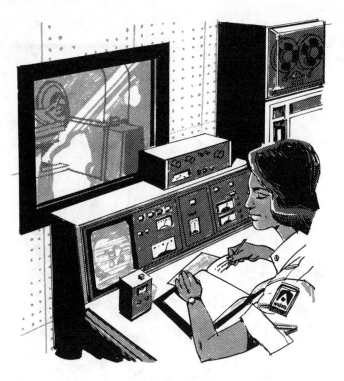

Technologist operating CAT scanner.

Who Will Do the CAT Scan?

The CAT scan will be done by a highly trained team of radiological technologists, technicians, and a radiologist. The **radiologist** is a physician who has very specialized training in radiation, ultrasound, scanning, and in making medical diagnoses.

Can CAT Scans Be Done on an Outpatient?

Yes. CAT scans lend themselves nicely for the outpatient. The procedure usually has no initial preparation and requires only that you lie still during the procedure.

How Long Does the Procedure Take?

This is difficult to answer, due to the varied types of studies done. The average time of a scan is about an hour.

Are There Any Complications or Side Effects to This Procedure?

As in any procedure, there is always a small chance for a side effect to occur. In this study, if contrast media (dye) is used, hives, sneezing, or other allergic reactions may occur.

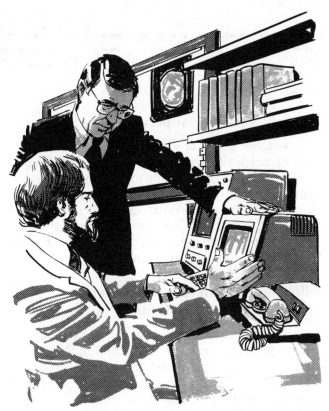

Radiologist making diagnosis from CAT scan.

Will the Procedure Be Covered by My Insurance?

Most insurance companies will pay the majority of the cost as well as the cost of the physician. The amount will differ from one insurance company to another.

Comments and Questions

Your Guide to Angiography

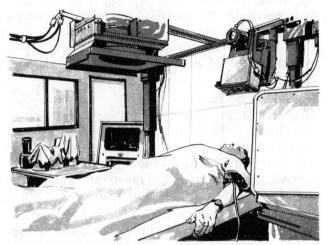

Special procedure room for angiography.

Introduction

Your doctor has ordered a special X-ray study or test for you. It is called an angiogram. An **angiogram** is the study of one or more blood vessels in your body. Dye is put into the blood vessels so they can be seen by X-ray. These pictures are recorded on X-ray film or movie film. It is very important that you understand the test because we will need your help. An angiogram may be done on any organ in any part of the body. If the doctor is going to study arteries, the test may be called an **arteriogram**. If the doctor is going to study veins, the test may be called a **venogram**. Both arteriograms and venograms are angiograms.

Why Is the Procedure Done?

Your doctor has probably told you why the test was ordered and what will be studied.

How Are Angiograms Named?

Angiograms are named for the area being studied. Below is a list of frequently done angiograms. Remember, the blood vessels studied may be arteries, veins, or both.
- Cerebral Angiograms—Head
- Carotid Angiograms—Neck
- Pulmonary Angiograms—Lungs
- Cardiac Angiograms—Heart
- Renal Angiograms—Kidneys
- Adrenal Angiograms—Adrenal, Glands
- Femoral Angiograms—Legs

- Brachial Angiograms—Arms
- Lymphatic Angiograms—Lymph Glands
- Mesenteric Angiograms—Mesentary Vessels (Stomach)
- Pancreatic Angiograms—Pancreas
- Spleenic Angiograms—Spleen
- Hepatic Angiograms—Liver

Who Will Do the Procedure?

The procedure will be done by a radiologist or a physician who specializes in this area. A **radiologist** is a physician who specializes in all types of X-ray procedures.

Where Will the Procedure Be Done?

The procedure will be done in a very special room in X-ray. When you are taken to the room, you will see a lot of equipment. The X-ray table is hard, but you will be made as comfortable as possible. The X-ray machine may look like a big "C." It may take normal X-ray pictures as well as movies.

How Is the Procedure Done?

Preparation for the Procedure
Usually you will not be given anything to eat or drink the night before the test. If your test

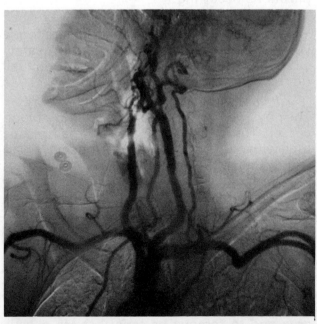

Angiogram of the aorta (aortagram). (By permission of the Radiology Dept., Lexington County Hospital, West Columbia, SC.)

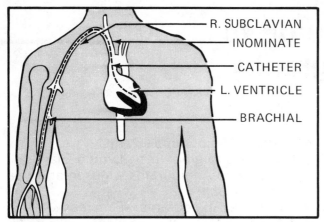

R. SUBCLAVIAN
INOMINATE
CATHETER
L. VENTRICLE
BRACHIAL

Brachial artery approach.

is scheduled later in the day, you may be given a light breakfast. Your doctor may give you a sleeping pill to help you sleep the night before the test. Just before you go to the X-ray department, the nurse may give you a shot to help you relax. You may want to use the bathroom before the shot is given since you will be in the X-ray department for a while.

How Long Does the Test Take?
This is very difficult to answer. The average time is about an hour, but depending on the pictures and other factors, it can be longer or shorter.

Why Can't I be Put to Sleep?
There will be times during the study when it will be necessary for you to hold your breath, move, not move, etc. Also, every time that you are given anesthesia, there is a chance of complications occurring.

Continuing with the Study
When you arrive in the special procedure room, you will be moved to the X-ray table. A safety strap may be put around you so you won't fall off the X-ray table.

Insertion of the Catheter!
The physician will insert a catheter into a blood vessel. The **catheter** is a very small plastic tube with one or more holes in it. The physician will decide whether to insert the special catheter through your arm (brachial approach), or through your leg (femoral approach). The area of entry in your leg is in the groin and is the most common site of entry. The next step is to make sure the area to be entered is clean and free of hair that may harbor germs. This is called **prepping** the insertion site. (The area may be shaved the night before the procedure.) An iodine solution is used to wash the area and to remove bacteria that are always present on the skin. The next step is to cover the area with sterile towels or sheets. These

towels and sheets are germ-free. This is done to prevent the chance of developing an infection. IT IS VERY IMPORTANT THAT YOU DO NOT TOUCH ANY OF THESE TOWELS OR SHEETS. Now we are ready to begin the procedure. The doctor will inject novocaine around the area. This will feel like a bee sting. It is like the medicine the dentist uses when working on your teeth. The area will become numb. You may feel the doctor pushing down, but you should not feel any pain. If you do, tell the doctor.

Will I be Cut?
No! To get the catheter into the blood vessel, the doctor will insert a needle into the skin. Then a wire will be put into the needle. The needle is removed and the catheter is put over the wire. Then the wire is removed, leaving the catheter inside the blood vessel.

Will Moving the Catheter be Painful?
No! Once the catheter is inside the blood vessel, you will not feel it. There are no nerves in the blood vessels. The doctor will position the catheter with the aid of **fluoroscopy**, a type of X-ray that lets the doctor see the catheter. After the catheter has been placed, the doctor may take some dye and test the position. You may have a warm feeling, but not pain.

The Angiogram!
We are now ready to take the pictures. The doctor will connect the catheter to a **dye injector**. This is a machine that delivers the dye at the right speed and the right amount. When the dye is injected, you may feel a very warm

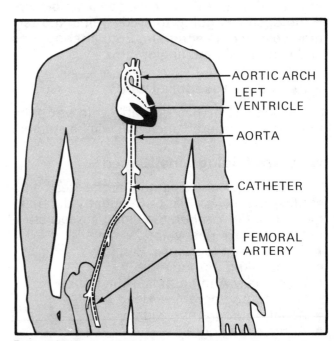

AORTIC ARCH
LEFT VENTRICLE
AORTA
CATHETER
FEMORAL ARTERY

Femoral artery approach.

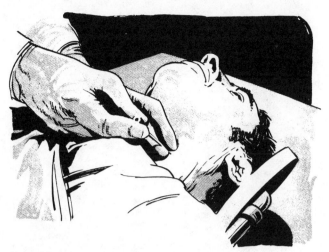

Carotid artery approach.

feeling. It is similar to stepping into a hot shower. This hot feeling will last only 10 seconds. Some women say that their feet and hands get hot. Some men say they can feel the warmth in their scrotum. Both men and women say that they feel like they are voiding (passing water). You are not. It is just a normal reaction. The dye makes you feel warm by dilating (opening) all of your blood vessels. *The most important part of the procedure now is that you do NOT move!* If you move, the pictures may have to be done again.

Additional Studies!

The doctor may wish to move the catheter and take another picture. This does not mean that you did something wrong, or that something is wrong with you. The doctor may want to see the blood vessel at a different angle, or perhaps a branch of the main artery or vein.

Post Procedure

When the doctor is satisfied with the pictures, the catheter will be removed. Pressure on the area for five to ten minutes prevents bleeding from the insertion site so the small hole from the catheter will close. This is the first step in scab formation. It is very similar to the healing of a cut finger.

Back to Your Room

When you return to your room, you will be requested to stay in bed for four to eight hours. This will allow the area to heal and you to rest. This does not mean get up and go to the bathroom. It means stay in bed. A nurse will be checking you very frequently for the first few hours. This is normal procedure. Your leg or arm, and your vital signs will be checked. If you are uncomfortable, ask for something for pain. It is very important that the nurse knows when you void (pass water). Please ring your bell and tell the nurse. If a family member takes

the bedpan or urinal from you, ask him or her to set it in the bathroom. *Do not empty it.* The urine will have to be measured.

When Will I Know the Results?

This is perhaps the most frequently asked question. Your physician will tell you the results of your tests later that day or early the next day. The films have to be read and any other data compiled during the test will have to be studied. Please have patience. The doctor knows how anxious you are for the test results, but wants to be able to give you complete answers to all of your questions.

Comments and Questions

Your Guide to Radiation Therapy

What Is Radiation Therapy

Radiation therapy is the use of X-rays, cobalt, linear accelerators, implants, and other sources of radiation to treat specific human diseases (e.g., cancer).

Who Receives Radiation Therapy?

The most common use of radiation therapy is for the management and treatment of cancer. It may be used alone or in combination with chemotherapy and surgical intervention.

Where Will It Be Done?

Radiation therapy is done in very specialized areas of a hospital or clinic. The radiation therapy unit is usually found near the X-ray department. The room is equipped with special safety features to protect you and the staff.

When Will It Be Done?

Radiation therapy will begin after preliminary tests that are done by your doctor. These may include blood studies, X-rays, etc. There will be a consultation between you, your doctor, and a specialized physician who will plan and follow you through your radiation treatments.

Who Will Give the Treatments?

Once radiation therapy has been decided upon, you will be sent to see a **radiation therapist,** a doctor who specializes in the use of radiation for treatment of disease. The doctor will carefully examine you, your X-rays, special tests, and records. If it is agreed that radiation treatment will help you, an individualized or personalized plan of treatment will be made. The doctor will ask you to sign a consent for treatment form called a **release**.

The **team approach** involves your own phyisican, a radiation therapist, a radiation physicist, nurses, and assistants.

Why Are More Tests Needed?

Before you actually start treatment, there will be a lot of planning and perhaps more tests done to make sure that you receive the very best care possible. One of the first steps will be to localize the area to be treated. This is done with the aid of CAT scans, X-rays, or ultrasound. It is important to know how big and how deep the cancer is. Radiation therapy not only kills cancer cells, but it also can harm normal cells, so this is a very important step. The physician will mark the area to be treated on your skin using a pen or some type of dye. It is important that this is not washed off.

The next step is planning what type of radiation will be used, how much, and for how long. Today, many of these figures are calculated with the aid of a computer. Another member of the health team, a **radiation physicist,** may help with this important part of planning your treatment.

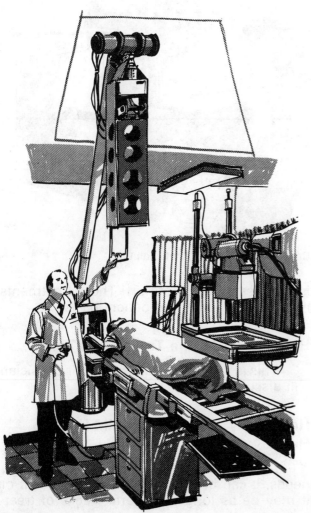

Radiation therapy room.

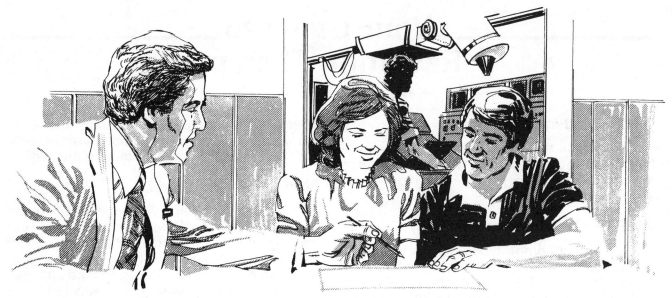

Therapist discussing radiation treatment with patient.

Procedure

Your radiation therapist will decide which treatment is best for you.

The receptionist will make an appointment for your treatments. You will be taken into a room with a very large machine and placed on a table. The assistants and physician will help you into the right position. They may have to use tape, pillows, etc. to keep you in the right position. Many times they will cover the skin around the area to be treated with lead to protect it from the radiation. The treatment

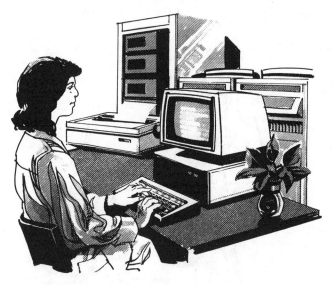

Calculating the amount of radiation.

is painless. It does not hurt! These treatments may be done on an outpatient basis.

How Long Will the Treatments Take?

This is very individualized. Your physician will discuss this with you.

How Many Treatments Will I Have to Have?

Again, this depends on your particular needs. It can be as short as one treatment or it may be as long as several weeks of treatments.

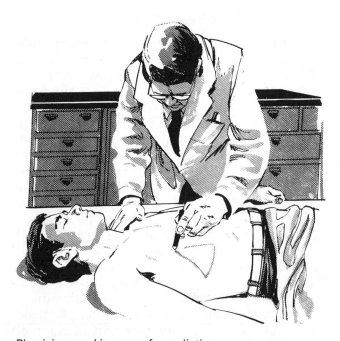

Physician marking area for radiation.

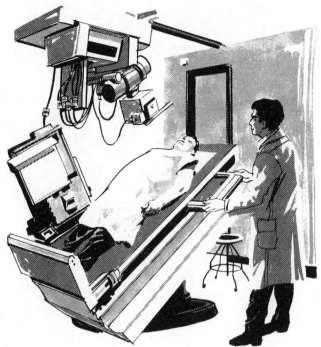

Positioning for radiation therapy.

Radioactive Implants:

The radiation therapist may decide the best way to treat your problem is to place radioactive material next to your skin. The implant is usually done under **anesthesia** (the area is numbed). The implant is then removed after one day to one week. While the implant is in your body, you will be placed in an **isolation room**. The number of visitors and the length of their stay will be limited. You will be taken out of isolation as soon as the implant is removed.

What Are the Complications of Radiation Therapy?

As with any type of procedure, there is always a chance of **complications** (side effects). Not all patients react the same to radiation therapy. If other therapies are going on simultaneously (chemotherapy or surgery), these may be a contributing factor to side effects. Most patients complete radiation therapy with minimal side effects.

Do I Have to Restrict My Activity During the Period of Treatment?

Your body is already weakened due to the disease, thus it is extremely important that you eat properly and get an adequate amount of sleep. You will be encouraged to continue with your normal activities as much as possible.

It is *very* important to protect the treatment site from sun, pressure, excessive heat (from hot water, heating pad, etc.), cold, injury from bumping, rubbing, etc. This area is already weakened from the disease plus the radiation treatments.

During radiation treatment, do not treat yourself for minor aches, pains, or injuries. *Notify your family physician and your radiation therapist before taking any medication or using any medical appliance.*

Will My Insurance Help to Cover the Cost of This Therapy?

Radiation therapy, like many other medical treatments, is expensive. Almost all insurance companies will cover not only the cost of the therapy, but also help with the professional charges of the physicians.

What Happens When I Finish the Therapy?

Follow-up care is an important part of the treatment program. You will be asked to see your family physician, as well as the radiation therapist. They will act as a team to assist you toward good health. When questions arise, write them down and ask your physician or radiation therapist to answer them.

Comments and Questions

2
Neurological Procedures

Electromyography and Nerve Conduction Studies (EMG)

An EMG is a graphic recording of the electrical potential across a muscle membrane. It is measured through a needle electrode.

An EMG is done to aid in the diagnosis of: (1) defects in transmission at neuromuscular junctions; (2) primary muscular disease; and (3) lower motor neuron disease. This test is helpful in diagnosis of poliomyelitis, parkinsonism, myasthenia gravis, amyotrophic lateral sclerosis, cord injuries, partial nerve injuries, and neuromuscular disorders.

Nurse's Responsibilities:
Pre-Test
1. Reassure patient.
2. Obtain permit.
3. Check chart to assess if patient is on any medication that may interfere with procedure:
   (a) muscle relaxants;
   (b) anticholinergics and cholinergics.

Precautions
Should not be done to patients who cannot cooperate.

Post-Procedure Care
If patient has pain:
1. Make him or her comfortable by applying warm compresses to areas where needles were inserted.
2. Give analgesics as ordered.
3. Resume previous orders.

Myography

Myography utilizes radiography and contrast media to visualize the spinal subarachnoid space. Myography is a neurologic procedure to diagnose spinal nerve root injury, tumors, herniated intervertebral disks which cause partial or complete blockage of the flow of cerebral spinal fluid, and arachnoiditis.

Nurse's Responsibilities:
Pre-Test
1. Food and fluids are restricted for 8 hours before the test. However, if the test is late in the day, clear liquids may be given for breakfast.

2. Be honest in patient preparation. Tell the patient he or she *may* feel pain on insertion of the needle. The patient may experience a warm or flushed feeling, nausea, vomiting, headache, or a salty taste on insertion of the dye, and discomfort or pain when placed in various positions during the procedure and/or removal of the dye.
3. Obtain a written permit.
4. Check chart and ask if patient is allergic to iodine, sea foods, or contrast media.
5. Administer pre-medications as ordered.

Precautions
1. Hypersensitivity to iodine.
2. Increased intracranial pressure.
3. Infection at puncture site.
4. Medication—tranquilizers (metrizoate contrast is not used).
5. Patient should be cooperative.

Post-Procedure Care
1. Make patient comfortable. Position will depend upon what type of contrast media was used in the procedure.
2. Monitor patient's neurologic status and vital signs as per order (usually q30 minutes X4, q1 hr X4, and then q4 hr).
3. Observe insertion site for any signs of CSF drainage, redness, hematoma, and swelling.
4. Encourage the patient to drink an increased amount of fluids.
5. Note amount and time of urination post procedure.
6. If patient experiences back pain, headache, radicular pain, or other signs of meningeal irritation, notify physician, keep patient quiet, and provide analgesics as per order.

Spinal Puncture (L.P.)

A lumbar puncture is usually done to obtain CSF for laboratory analysis. The analysis of this fluid is valuable in the diagnosis of viral or bacterial meningitis, CSF blockage or obstruction, tumors, intracranial hemmorhage, infections, abscesses, and other central nervous system disorders.

Two other important reasons for doing a lumbar puncture are to measure the CSF pressures and to instill medications.

Nurse's Responsibilities:

Pre-Test
1. Explain procedure to the patient and family. Explain the necessity of holding still.
2. Food and fluid usually are not restricted before the procedure.
3. Obtain a written permit.
4. Administer pre-medications as per order.

Precautions
1. Extreme caution should be used in the patient with elevated intracranial pressure.
2. Additional personnel will be needed if the patient is uncooperative.
3. Procedure is contraindicated if there is an infection on or near the insertion site.

Post-Procedure Care
1. Make patient comfortable. Check orders to see if head of bed may be elevated 30°.
2. Monitor neurologic status and vital signs q15 min X4, q30 min X4, q1 hr X4, and then q4 hr.
3. Observe insertion site for any signs of CSF drainage, redness, or swelling.
4. Encourage the patient to drink an increased amount of fluids.
5. Note amount and time of urination post procedure.
6. If patient experiences headache, back pain, radicular pain, or other signs of meningeal irritation, notify physician, keep patient quiet, and administer analgesics as per order.

Electroencephalography

Electroencephalography is the graphic representation of electrical activity in the brain. These electrical waves are picked up by electrodes placed on the scalp. The signal is then transmitted to the electroencephalograph, where the signal is amplified and recorded on paper.

This procedure is done to assess the presence and type of seizure disorders (epilepsy); to aid in the diagnosis of tumors, abscesses, and other intracranial lesions; to confirm brain death; and to evaluate brain activity in central nervous system infections, psychological disorders, trauma, metabolic disorders, and in mental retardation.

Nurse's Responsibilities:

Pre-Test
1. Explain the procedure to the patient.
2. Reassure that the patient will not be shocked.
3. Be sure the patient eats before the test—hypoglycemia may change the brain wave pattern.
4. Physician may ask that the patient refrain from smoking or drinking coffee or cola before the procedure.
5. If a sleeping EEG is to be done, the patient should be kept awake the night before the procedure.
6. Administer pre-medication as per order.
7. Note any medications the patient has taken that may interfer with the procedure.

Precautions
1. Observe patient for signs and symptoms of seizure activity.

Post-Procedure Care
1. Make patient comfortable. Assist in the removal of electrode paste from hair.
2. Observe patient for seizure activity.
3. Resume previous orders.

Your Guide to Electromyography & Nerve Conduction Study

Introduction

Your physician has ordered a special examination or test called an electromyogram or EMG. This information will discuss many of the questions you may have concerning the test.

What is an EMG?

An **EMG** is a method of recording the electrical activity of selected muscles at rest and during exercise through a needle electrode.

What Is a Nerve Conduction Study?

The nerve conduction study is a separate part of the electromyography procedure. The **nerve conduction study** is the recorded conduction measured from the time the nerve is stimulated until there is a detected response.

Why Is an EMG Done?

An EMG is done to aid in the diagnosis of primary and secondary muscular and neuro-muscular diseases.

Why Is a Nerve Conduction Study Done?

A nerve conduction study is done to aid in the diagnosis of diseases and injuries of the peripheral nervous system.

Is There Any Preparation for an EMG?

No! This test may be done on an out-patient or an in-patient basis. It may be scheduled at any time of the day without regard to whether the patient has or has not eaten. Some physicians may restrict cola, coffee, or cigarettes 2 to 4 hours prior to the test.

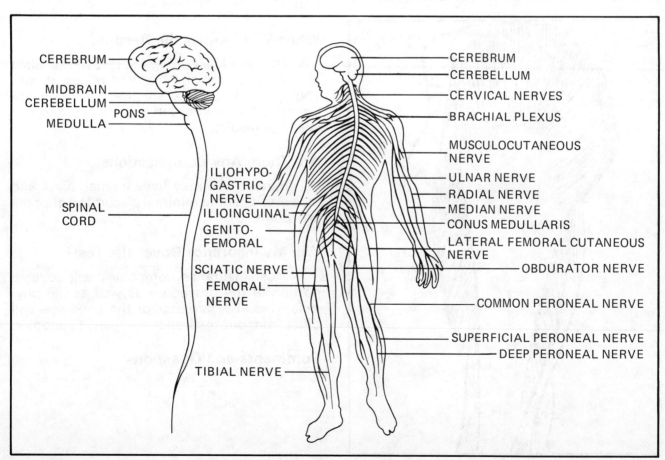

The central nervous system.

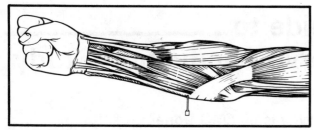

Needle insertion into the arm muscles.

Where Is the Procedure Done?

The EMG procedure may be done in any one of a number of areas: a physician's office, hospital, or a clinic.

Who Will do the Procedure?

The EMG is done under the direction of a neurologist, but may be done by an EMG technician. A **neurologist** is a doctor who specializes in the study of nerve and muscular disease. Other qualified physicians, such as those specializing in physical therapy, may also do this procedure.

How is the Procedure Done?

You will be taken into a procedure room or office and placed on a table where you will be made as comfortable as possible. The area or region of the body to be tested will be exposed. (You may be asked to put on a hospital gown.) The physician will turn on a type of recording instrument called a **myograph**, and will connect a ground wire and a special type of needle to the machine. The needle is very small in diameter and about ¾ inches long. The needle is inserted very carefully and quickly into the muscle. A metal plate called a **reference electrode** is attached to the skin, or placed under you. The electrical activity is noted at several areas of the body. It is not painful, but may be uncomfortable. This electrical activity may be seen on a type of television called an **oscilloscope**, as well as heard as the electrical activity is converted into sound waves.

How Is a Nerve Conduction Study Done?

A nerve is stimulated through the skin by an electrical impulse and its response is measured by a reference electrode at a distance from the stimulated nerve.

How Long Will It Take?

The average length of time is about one hour.

When Will I Know the Results?

The physician doing the test will tabulate all the data from the test and review it with your physician, who will then make an appointment with you and your family and discuss the results.

Are There Any Complications?

Rarely! You may have a small black and blue area or some minimal discomfort after the procedure.

Will My Insurance Cover the Test?

Most insurance companies will cover a portion of the procedure as well as the physician fee. The amount of the coverage will differ from one insurance company to another.

Comments and Questions

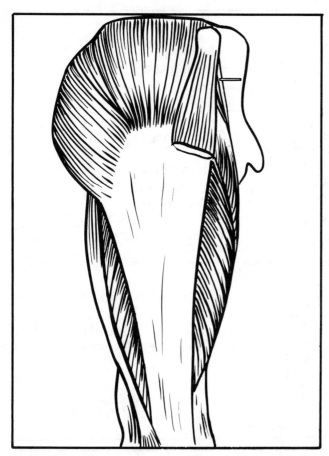

Needle insertion into the leg muscles.

Your Guide to
Myelography

Introduction

Your doctor has ordered a special examination called a myelogram. This information will discuss many of the questions you may have concerning this test.

What Is a Myelogram?

A **myelogram** is a special X-ray of the spinal cord. It is possible *only* because the doctor can inject dye into the spinal canal. This dye outlines the spinal cord. The spinal canal is a tube full of cerebrospinal fluid that runs through the **vertebrae** or spinal column (backbones).

IMPORTANT:—tell the physician if you are allergic to iodine or shellfish.

Why Is a Myelogram Done?

A myelogram is done to help in the diagnosis of diseases of the central nervous system or damage of the vertebrae.

Is There Any Special Preparation for a Myelogram?

You will be asked not to eat or drink anything after midnight of the day of your procedure. This is called **N.P.O.** (nothing by mouth). A nurse will remind you of this, and will remove any fluid just prior to this time. If your procedure is to be scheduled late in the afternoon, you may be given a clear breakfast and then the fluids will be removed.

Your doctor will order some medication to help you relax just prior to being taken to the X-ray department.

Where Will the Procedure Be Done?

Myelograms are usually done in the X-ray special procedure room in the department of radiology (X-ray department).

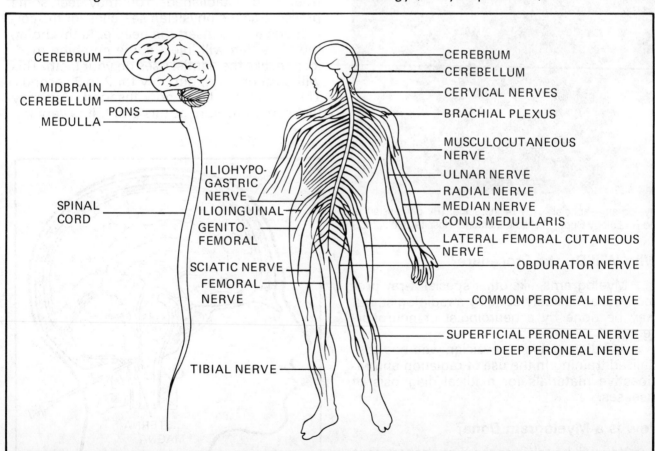

CEREBRUM
MIDBRAIN
CEREBELLUM
PONS
MEDULLA
SPINAL CORD
ILIOHYPO-GASTRIC NERVE
ILIOINGUINAL
GENITO-FEMORAL
SCIATIC NERVE
FEMORAL NERVE
TIBIAL NERVE

CEREBRUM
CEREBELLUM
CERVICAL NERVES
BRACHIAL PLEXUS
MUSCULOCUTANEOUS NERVE
ULNAR NERVE
RADIAL NERVE
MEDIAN NERVE
CONUS MEDULLARIS
LATERAL FEMORAL CUTANEOUS NERVE
OBDURATOR NERVE
COMMON PERONEAL NERVE
SUPERFICIAL PERONEAL NERVE
DEEP PERONEAL NERVE

The central nervous system.

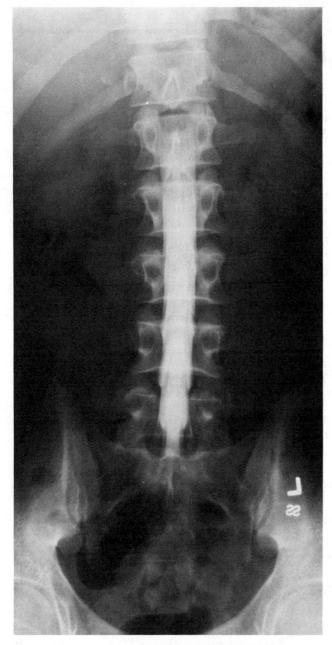

Myelogram—special X-ray of the spine. (By permission of the Radiology Dept., Richland Memorial Hospital, Cola, SC.)

Who Will Do the Procedure?

Myelograms, like other special X-ray procedures, are usually done by a radiologist, but may be done by a neurologist or neurosurgeon.

A **radiologist** is a physician who has specialized training in the use of radiation and radioactive materials for medical diagnosis of diseases.

How Is a Myelogram Done?

You will be taken to the X-ray department and placed on a special table that will be moved

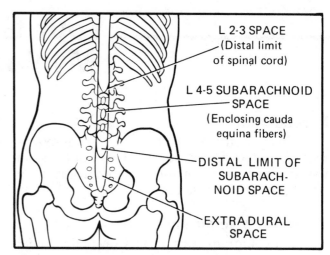

Lumbar approach for needle insertion.

up and down. The medical team will help to position you. Your vital signs will be measured and monitored throughout the test. The most common position is **prone** (face down), with a pillow under your hips (lumbar approach). This position promotes an easy entry into the spinal space. An alternate method is a **cisternal approach**. The needle is inserted at the base of the head. The area is cleaned and a sterile (germ-free) field established. You may feel some pressure as the physician searches for the correct position to insert the needle. At this point, the physician will inject some numbing medication, like the dentist uses on your teeth. This will burn or sting, but only for 2 to 3 seconds. The spinal needle is now inserted. You may feel some pressure at this point. It is very im-

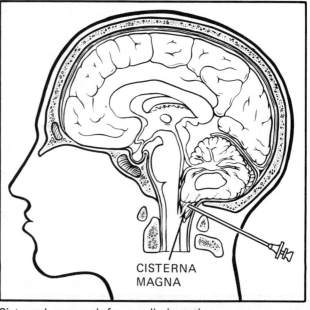

Cisternal approach for needle insertion.

portant that you do not move. Some cerebro-spinal fluid is removed and contrast media (dye) is inserted via the spinal needle. You may feel flushed or warm when the dye is injected.

It is at this point that X-ray pictures are taken. The X-ray table will be moved in different positions. You will not fall! It is important that you do what the physician and X-ray technologists ask you to do!

When the test is complete, the dye will be removed, and the needle will be withdrawn. A new dye, which is now being used, does not have to be removed. The area will be cleaned and covered with a bandaid.

When you return to your room, you will be asked to lie flat for 8 to 24 hours, and encouraged to drink fluids.

How Long Does the Test Take?

Everyone is a little different. The average time is about an hour.

When Will I Know the Results?

Your physician will tell you the results as soon as he or she has seen the pictures, and conferred with the physician who did the procedure.

Are There Any Complications or Side Effects?

As in any procedure, there is always a risk of complication. However, the benefit from the information gained from the test far outweighs the risk. The two most common side effects are headache and backache.

Will My Insurance Cover This Procedure?

Most insurance companies will cover the procedure and physician fee. The amount of coverage will vary from company to company.

27

Your Guide to Spinal (Lumbar) Puncture

Introduction

Your physician has requested that you have a special test called a lumbar puncture (LP). This information will discuss many of the questions you may have concerning the test. This test may be referred to as a spinal tap or an LP.

What Is a Lumbar Puncture?

A **lumbar puncture** is the introduction of a needle into a space of the spinal canal. The **spinal canal** is a tube full of cerebrospinal fluid, which runs through the **vertebrae** or spinal column (backbones).

Why Is a Lumbar Puncture Done?

A lumbar puncture is done to obtain information about the cerebrospinal fluid (CSF), CSF pressure, or to inject medication directly into the spinal canal. This information can then be used to aid in the diagnosis, assessment, and treatment of diseases involving the central nervous system.

Is There Any Preparation for the Procedure?

Lumbar punctures are often done as an emergency procedure. However, if this test is scheduled, food may be withheld until the test is over. This test may be done on an out-patient basis, but more often is done as an in-patient procedure.

Where is the Procedure Done?

A lumbar puncture may be done at a patient's bedside or in any number of locations in the hospital. Some of these areas may be the emergency room, X-ray department, operating room, specialty units, etc.

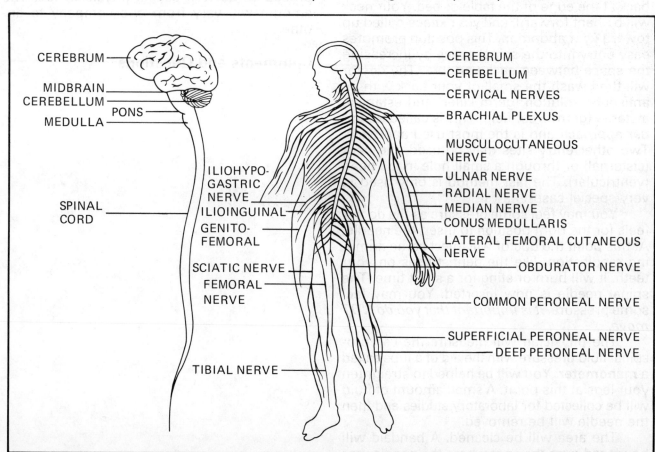

CEREBRUM

MIDBRAIN
CEREBELLUM
PONS
MEDULLA

SPINAL CORD

ILIOHYPO-GASTRIC NERVE
ILIOINGUINAL
GENITO-FEMORAL

SCIATIC NERVE
FEMORAL NERVE

TIBIAL NERVE

CEREBRUM
CEREBELLUM
CERVICAL NERVES
BRACHIAL PLEXUS
MUSCULOCUTANEOUS NERVE
ULNAR NERVE
RADIAL NERVE
MEDIAN NERVE
CONUS MEDULLARIS
LATERAL FEMORAL CUTANEOUS NERVE
OBDURATOR NERVE
COMMON PERONEAL NERVE
SUPERFICIAL PERONEAL NERVE
DEEP PERONEAL NERVE

The central nervous system.

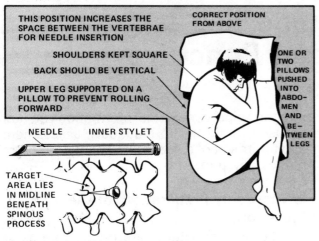

THIS POSITION INCREASES THE SPACE BETWEEN THE VERTEBRAE FOR NEEDLE INSERTION

CORRECT POSITION FROM ABOVE

SHOULDERS KEPT SQUARE

BACK SHOULD BE VERTICAL

UPPER LEG SUPPORTED ON A PILLOW TO PREVENT ROLLING FORWARD

ONE OR TWO PILLOWS PUSHED INTO ABDOMEN AND BE- TWEEN LEGS

NEEDLE   INNER STYLET

TARGET AREA LIES IN MIDLINE BENEATH SPINOUS PROCESS

Position for needle insertion.

Who Will Perform the Procedure?

A physician who has had special training will do the procedure.

How Is the Procedure Done?

A nurse or other member of the medical team will help you get positioned for the test. You will be asked to lie on your side with your back at the edge of the table or bed. Your neck will be bent forward, and your knees pulled up toward your abdomen. This position promotes easy entry into the spinal space by increasing the space between each vertebra. The doctor will then wash the small of your back with an antiseptic solution (germ killer) and establish a sterile (germ-free) field. This is called a **lumbar approach** and is the most used approach. Two other entry sites may be used, the neck (cisternal) or through a small hole in the head (ventricular). The last method is only used in very special cases.

You may feel some pressure as the doctor feels for the right position to insert the needle. At this point the doctor will inject some numbing medication, like the dentist uses on your teeth. It will burn or sting for a short time. The spinal needle is now inserted. You may feel some pressure. *It is important that you do NOT move.*

The physician will measure the cerebrospinal fluid pressure with the aid of a tube called a **manometer**. You will be helped to straighten your legs at this point. A small amount of fluid will be collected for laboratory studies and then the needle will be removed.

The area will be cleaned. A bandaid will be placed over the spot where the needle was removed.

After the procedure, you will be asked to lie flat in bed for four to twelve hours and will be encouraged to drink fluids.

How Long Does the Test Take?

The average time is about 15 to 30 minutes starting when the doctor arrives.

When Will I Know the Results?

Your doctor will tell you the results as soon as possible. There may be some delay while the laboratory tests are being done.

Are There Any Complications or Side Effects?

As in any procedure, there are always some risks. However, the information gained from such a test far outweighs any risk. The most common side effects are some local discomfort and headache, which go away within a few hours.

Will My Insurance Cover This Procedure?

Most insurance companies will cover the procedure as well as the physician fee. The amount will vary from one company to another.

Comments and Questions

Your Guide to Electroencephalography (EEG)

Introduction

Your doctor has ordered a special test for you called an electroencephalogram or EEG.

What Is an EEG?

Stated simply, an **EEG** is a graphic record of the brain waves.

Why Is an EEG Done?

An EEG is done to identify and assess the type and amount of electrical activity in a particular area of the brain. This information may then be used to determine medical treatment. The EEG may be done while you are awake or asleep.

Is There Any Preparation for the Test?

Yes!
1. On the evening prior to your test, you may be requested to stay up an hour or two later than usual.
2. The morning of your test, you may be asked to awaken earlier than normal (5 or 6 a.m.).
3. It is very important, if your test is not scheduled until later in the day, that you *do not* take a nap before your test.

4. When you are ready for your test, be sure you remove all hairpins, clips, wigs, etc.

Where Is the Test Done?

EEGs may be done in several areas of the hospital. Some of these areas may include the critical care unit, bedside, EEG department, treatment areas, and operating room.

Who Will Do the Test?

The actual procedure will be done by a highly trained technician, who will then give the data obtained from the procedure to a neurologist. A **neurologist** is a physician who specializes in neuro-muscular disorders.

How Is the Procedure Done?

You will be taken to the area where the procedure is to be done, and made comfortable in a bed.

If you are taking any medication, tell the technician so he or she may make a note of it. (Some medications will affect the brain wave patterns.)

The technician will carefully part off your hair and place cream and then electrodes on

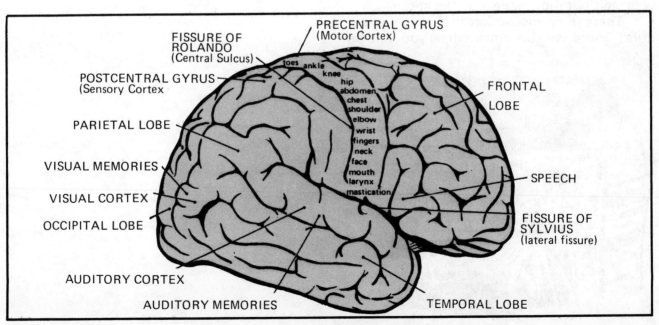

Diagram of the brain.

front-central

L

R

central-occipital

L

R

frontal-temporal

L

R

temporal-occipital

L

R

| 50 µV
|_____
1 second

EEG tracing.

your scalp. The **electrodes** are the means of measuring the electrical activity of the brain at the scalp surface. The cream will not damage your hair but may leave it a little sticky.

There is *no* discomfort during the procedure! There will be times when you will be given specific things to do. These may include deep breaths, opening and closing your eyes, etc. At some point in the study, the technician will request that you try to sleep.

When enough information is gathered, you will be awakened and the wires and cream removed from your scalp.

You will then be taken back to your room. If this was done on an out-patient basis, you may leave the hospital.

How Long Does the Procedure Take?

The time will vary from one patient to another, but the average time is 1 to 3 hours.

When Will I Know the Results?

When all of the data is tabulated, your physician will tell you the results.

Are There Any Complications or Side Effects?

No!

Will My Insurance Cover This Procedure?

Most insurance companies will cover the procedure as well as the physician fee. The amount of coverage will vary from company to company.

Comments and Questions

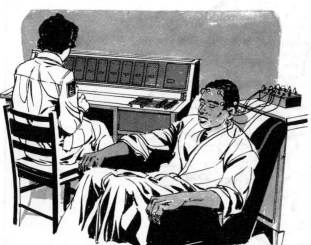

Patient connected to EEG machine.

3

Cardiology Studies

Non-Invasive Cardiology Studies

Another very appropriate title for this group of studies would be graphic recording studies. This group of studies has six subdivisions: electrocardiography, Holter and telemetry monitoring, stress testing electrocardiography, echocardiography, phonocardiography, and vectorcardiography.

Each of the above groups will be defined and their individual purposes will be briefly discussed.

The nurses' responsibilities are similar in all of these studies and will be discussed as a single topic.

ELECTROCARDIOGRAPHY (ECG)
An ECG is the graphic recording of the heart's electrical activity. It is generated by the conduction system of the heart.

Purpose:
  a. To aid in the diagnosis of cardiac dysrhythmias, cardiac conduction abnormalities, infectious processes, trauma, acute myocardial infarctions, ischemia, cardiac hypertrophy, and electrolyte disturbances.
  b. To help assess the size and the extent of a myocardial infarction.
  c. To monitor the recovery period of a myocardial infarct.
  d. To evaluate the effectiveness of drug therapies and/or surgical intervention.

HOLTER AND TELEMETRY MONITORING
Holter monitoring is a continuous ECG tracing (one lead) recorded on tape for a specified amount of time (8 to 24 hours is normal). It is recorded as the patient does daily living tasks. The patient wears the whole recording device. This may be done as an out-patient.

Telemetry monitoring is the transmission of information (ECG tracing—single lead) via an electronic device. Patient is usually monitored over a two to three day period of time. As above, the patient wears the transmitter, but not the recorder. This is only done on patients within specified distance from the nurses station.

Purpose of both procedures:
  a. To aid in the diagnosis of cardiac dysrhythmias.
  b. To evaluate drug therapy.
  c. To evaluate pacemaker therapy.
  d. To follow the course of a myocardial infarction.
  e. To evaluate the patient with chest pain, dyspnea, syncopy, etc.

STRESS EXERCISE ELECTROCARDIOGRAPHY
A stress ECG is the graphic recording of the heart's electrical activity at rest and during exercise.

Purpose:
  a. To evaluate the heart with an increased oxygen demand.
  b. To aid in the diagnosis of chest pain.
  c. As a post-procedure function test for the patient who underwent cardiac surgery.
  d. To evaluate patients who are potential cardiac risks due to age, heredity, etc.
  e. To assist in the establishment of an exercise program.
  f. To evaluate drug and/or surgical therapy.

ECHOCARDIOGRAPHY
An echocardiogram is an ultrasonic procedure that records the size, wall motion, and composition of the heart and great vessels by the use of a transducer.

Purpose:
  a. To evaluate size of the heart and aid in diagnosis of cardiomyopathies and cardiac hypertrophy.
  b. To aid in the diagnosis of vascular abnormalities of the great vessels and heart.
  c. To evaluate cardiac function.
  d. To aid in the diagnosis of valvular disease.
  e. To assist in the diagnosis of pericardial effusion.
  f. To detect atrial myxomas.

PHONOCARDIOGRAPHY
A phonocardiogram is the actual recording of heart sounds with the use of microphones.

Purpose:
  a. To aid in the identification of heart sounds with precise timing of cardiac events.
  b. To assist in the calculation of systolic time intervals.
  c. To assist in the diagnosis of valvular disease, ventricular enlargement, ischemia, or infarction and pericarditis.

VECTORCARDIOGRAPHY
A vectorcardiogram is a procedure used to detect muscular abnormalities by measuring the magnitude and direction of the heart's action currents. This is done by the use of two simultaneous leads.

Purpose:
  a. To aid in diagnosis of myocardial infarction.
  b. To detect hypertrophy (ventricular).
  c. To assist in evaluation of *interventricular* conduction disturbances.

d. To add further information and clarification of electrocardiograms.

Nurse's Responsibilities:

Pre-Test
1. Explain procedure to patient. (All of these procedures may be done on an out-patient basis.)
2. Have patient put on a hospital gown.
3. If test is to be done in patient's room, assist technologist in patient positioning.

Precautions
1. Patient should be cooperative.
2. Ensure there are *no* electrical hazards.

Post-Procedure Care
1. Make patient comfortable.
2. Assist patient in removing any gel or tape left post procedures.

Cardiac Electrophysiology Studies

A cardiac electrophysiology study graphically records the electrical physiological function of the heart. This is accomplished through special pacing catheters attached to a recorder.

The cardiac electrophysiology study is done to determine if there is a conduction dysfunction and where this dysfunction is located (re-entry accessory pathway, ectopic foci, dysrhythmia, evaluation of drug or pacing therapy, etc.).

Nurse's Responsibilities

Pre-Test
1. Explain the procedure to the patient and family. This is often done by the physician but the patient and family may need reinforcement.
2. Check to see if a permit has been signed. If not, have one signed and witnessed.
3. Some physicians may prefer that their patients are NPO for the test. This is especially true if elective cardioversion or drug challenge is to be part of the procedure.
4. The patient should be in a hospital gown.
5. If an IV has not been started, start one with an 18g jelco or other catheter. This is to be used as a fluid line or for drug administration.
6. Have the patient void prior to the procedure.
7. Prepare patient and chart for transfer to the electrophysiology lab or special procedure area.
8. On call to the lab, give pre-operative medication as per order.

Precautions
1. Check to see if patient has a prolonged coagulation time.
2. Patient should be cooperative and be able to lie still for 1 to 2 hours.
3. Check the medications the patient is on and list them on the front of the chart.

4. Note if the patient has a special medical problem (diabetes, epilepsy, etc.).
5. Emergency equipment and medications should be available for use.

Post-Procedure Care
1. Monitor patient's vital signs and heart rhythm post study.
2. Make patient comfortable and check insertion site for bleeding or hematoma.
3. Warm compresses to area of insertion are often soothing.
4. Check the IV site for signs of infiltration or withdrawn for hematoma.
5. Order meal tray or snack for patient.
6. Check chart for pertinent post-op orders.
7. Check peripheral pulses, color, and warmth of the extremity. (Compare with other extremity.)

Pacemakers

The pacemaker group is divided into two divisions: temporary pacemakers, which are utilized for emergency procedures; and permanent pacemakers, utilized for long-term therapy in abnormalities of the conduction system.

Both of these types of pacemakers have in common their two component parts: the *generator*, which is battery-operated, and the *pacing wire*, which is bipolar or unipolar. However, there is a difference in whether the generator is implanted (permanent pacemaker) or outside the body (temporary pacemaker).

The pacing wire is normally placed in the right ventricle for ventricular pacing, but may be inserted directly into the heart muscle. This latter procedure is known as an endocardial approach and is utilized most often during surgery. The pacing wire may be inserted into the right atrium for atrial pacing or an electrode from the same pacing wire is placed into the atria and ventricle for A-V sequential pacing.

Nurse's Responsibilities

These steps are needed for both the temporary and permanent pacemaker.

Pre-Test
1. Explain the procedure to the patient and family. If this has been done by the physician, the family and patient still may need some reassurance.
2. Ensure that a permit has been signed. If this is an emergency procedure, a family member may sign for the patient.
3. If an IV has not been started, start one with an 18g or larger needle. This will be used for fluids and/or medications.
4. The patient for a permanent pacemaker may be NPO for the procedure or on clear liquids if the procedure is performed late in the day.

5. Explain to the patient that he or she will be awake during the procedure, but will be made as comfortable as possible.
6. Ask patient to void prior to procedure.
7. Ask the patient to put on a hospital gown.
8. Prepare the patient and chart for transfer to the area where the procedure is to be done.
9. Pre-medicate patient on call for the procedure as per order.

Precautions
1. The patient should be cooperative. If the patient cannot cooperate, notify the pacemaker team.
2. The patient should be cardiac monitored to and from the procedure area.
3. It may be the nurse's responsibility to order the correct generator and wire for a permanent pacemaker.
4. Pre-existing medical problems should be noted on the front of the chart (diabetes, epilepsy, bleeding tendency, allergies, etc.).
5. The procedure area should be equipped with emergency equipment and medications.

Post-Procedure Care
1. Connect patient to cardiac monitor.
2. Monitor vital signs as per order.
3. Make patient comfortable and check insertion site for drainage, hematoma, etc.
4. Check chart to see what settings the pacemaker is set on.
5. If a temporary pacemaker has been inserted, check leads and generator to make sure it is covered and safe from falling.
6. Medicate patient with analgesics as per order for discomfort.
7. Check IV site for signs of infiltration.
8. Resume prior orders.

Cardiac Catheterization

Cardiac catheterization is an invasive diagnostic procedure to study the chamber, valves, and vascular system of the heart and great vessels. This is accomplished by passing a catheter into the venous system to study the right side of the heart or through the arterial system to study the left side of the heart.

This procedure is done: (1) to detect valve disease, congenital abnormalities, cardiac trauma, coronary stenosis, myocardial function; (2) to determine the etiology of chest pain; and (3) to assess drug therapy or post surgical therapy, etc.

Nurse's Responsibilities

Pre-Test
1. Explain the procedure to the patient and family. If this has been done by the physician, reinforce what has been said. Explain that during the study, upon receiving the dye, the patient will have an intense warm feeling, which will only last for a few seconds.

2. Ensure that a permit has been signed. If not, have one signed and witnessed.
3. Patient will be NPO post midnight for the procedure. Clear liquids may be given if case is scheduled late in the day.
4. Have patient put on a hospital gown.
5. Have patient void prior to going to the procedure room.
6. Question patient concerning an allergic reaction to contrast dye or shellfish.
7. Check IV for signs of infiltration. If patient does not have an IV, start one with an 18g or greater needle.
8. Check chart for recent blood studies and note on front of chart any pertinent pre-existing medical problems (diabetes, epilepsy, bleeding tendency, etc.).
9. Prepare the patient for transport.
10. Give pre-medication as per order on call.

Precautions
1. The contrast media used in cardiac catheterization is an iodine-based dye. Patients who are sensitive to iodine should be prepped with steroids if the test is necessary.
2. Patients should be cooperative. If the patient cannot cooperate, notify the catheterization team.
3. Contrast media is excreted via the kidneys. Extreme caution should be used in the patient with a compromised urinary system.
4. Laboratory should have emergency equipment and medications.

Post-Procedure Care
1. Patient usually is cardiac monitored for 24 hours post procedure.
2. Monitor vital signs q15 min X4, q30 min X4, q1 hr X4 and then q4 hr.
3. Observe insertion site for bleeding, swelling, or hematoma.
4. Check peripheral pulses with vital signs and note color and warmth of the extremity. (Compare with other extremity.)
5. Enforce complete bedrest for 8 to 24 hours or as per order.
6. Check IV for signs of infiltration.
7. Note time and amount when the patient first voids.
8. Review chart for pertinent orders.
9. Administer analgesics as per order for patient comfort.
10. If patient is not NPO, encourage fluids and order snack if meal time is passed.

Pericardiocentesis

The pericardiocentesis procedure is a needle aspiration of pericardial fluid from the pericardial sac surrounding the heart. This procedure can be either diagnostic or therapeutic.

Diagnostically, this procedure is done to obtain a sample of pericardial fluid for analysis to confirm or identify the reason for pericardial effusion. Therapeutically, this procedure may be done to relieve tension on the heart due to a large effusion from trauma or other reasons, or for the instillation of medications.

Pericardiocentesis may be done as an emergency procedure to relieve cardiac tamponade.

Nurse's Responsibilities

Pre-Test
1. Explain the procedure to patient and family.
2. Ensure that a permit has been signed. If this procedure is an emergency, a family member may sign the permit.
3. The patient normally can eat and drink prior to the test.
4. Have patient put on hospital gown.
5. If the patient does not have an IV, start one with an 18g or larger needle.
6. Prepare patient and chart for transport.
7. Give pre-medication on call as per order.

Precautions
1. The patient should be cooperative. If not, notify the physician.
2. Check the chart for recent blood studies and current antibiotic usage. Note these on the front of the chart.
3. Ensure that the ECG equipment and all other electrical equipment are properly grounded.
4. Observe ECG closely during procedure for ectopy and S-T changes.
5. Monitor patient's vital signs throughout procedure.
6. Ensure aspirated fluid is placed into proper containers and correctly labeled.

Post-Procedure Care
1. Patient should be cardiac monitored for 24 hours post procedure for dysrhythmias.
2. Check vital signs q15 min X4, q30 min X4, q1 hr X4, and then q4 hr.
3. Check insertion site for drainage.
4. Check IV for signs of infiltration.
5. Be aware that the patient may have respiratory or cardiac distress.

6. Administer analgesics as per order.

Elective Cardioversion

An elective cardioversion is usually done to terminate tachydysrhythmias. This is done to re-establish a normal rate and rhythm for the patient. It is accomplished through a synchronized, external direct current charge.

Nurse's Responsibilities

Pre-Test
1. Explain the procedure to the patient and family. The patient is usually very apprehensive. Give him or her time to verbalize fears.
2. Explain that the patient will be given medications so that he or she will not feel the shock.
3. Ensure that a permit has been signed.
4. If the patient does not have an IV, start one with an 18g or larger needle.
5. Have patient remove any dentures.
6. Have patient put on a hospital gown.
7. Food and fluids may be withheld until after the test.
8. Prepare patient and chart for transport to the procedure area.

Precautions
1. Ensure that the ECG and defibrillator are properly grounded.
2. Check IV for signs of infiltration.
3. Ensure defibrillator is in the synchronization mode.
4. Procedure area should be equipped with emergency equipment and medications.

Post-Procedure Care
1. Monitor vital signs closely until patient is fully responded.
2. Patient should be ECG monitored briefly post elective cardioversion to assess its effectiveness.
3. Place soothing cream over site where the paddles were placed.
4. When fully responsive, patient may eat and drink.
5. Check chart for pertinent medication orders.
6. Resume all other previous orders.

Your Guide to Non-Invasive Cardiology Studies

Introduction

Your doctor has ordered one or more non-invasive cardiology procedures to be done. This information will briefly discuss what each of these procedures are, and why and how they are done.

What Is an Electrocardiogram (ECG)?

An **ECG** is a graphic representation (picture) of the electrical activity of the heart.

What Is Holter and Telemetry Monitoring?

Holter monitoring is a continuous ECG tracing recorded on tape over a specified amount of time (4 to 24 hours). **Telemetry monitoring** is a continuous ECG tracing recorded at periodic intervals on paper over a given period of time.

What Is an Echocardiogram?

An **echocardiogram** is the use of ultrasound in recording the size, motion, and composition of the heart and great vessels.

What Is a Vectorcardiogram?

A **vectorcardiogram** is a graphic representation (picture) of the magnitude and direction of the heart's electrical force (action currents) in the form of a vector loop.

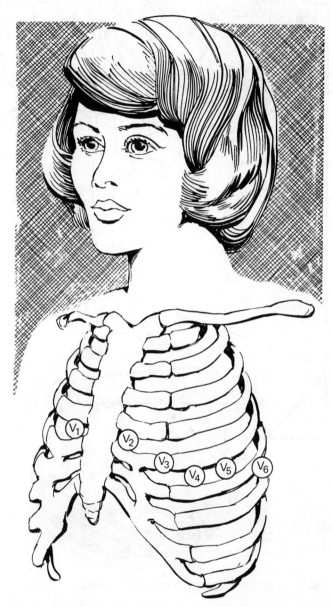

Placement of electrodes for an electrocardiogram.

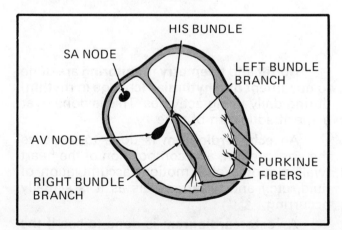

Electrical conduction system of the heart.

What Is a Stress Test?

A **cardiac stress test** is a graphic record of the resulting electrical activity of the heart during forced physical exertion.

What Is a Phonocardiogram?

A **phonocardiogram** is a graphic recording of the actual heart sounds.

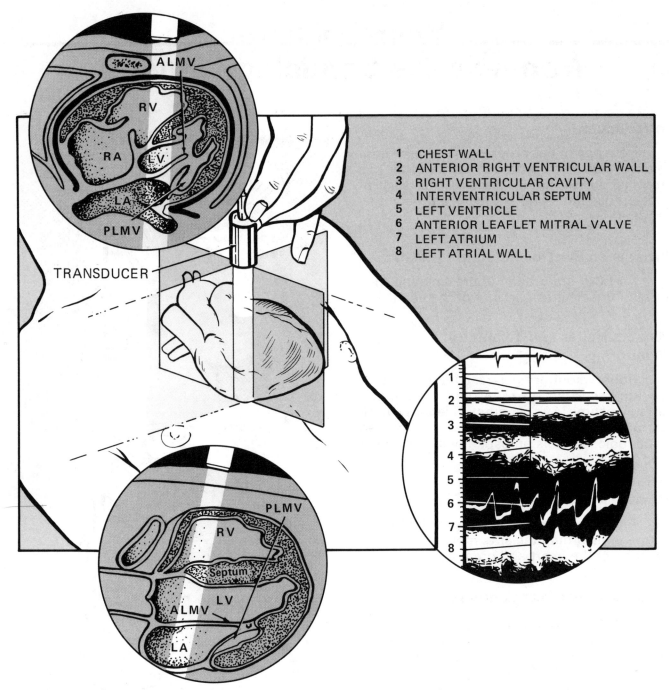

1 CHEST WALL
2 ANTERIOR RIGHT VENTRICULAR WALL
3 RIGHT VENTRICULAR CAVITY
4 INTERVENTRICULAR SEPTUM
5 LEFT VENTRICLE
6 ANTERIOR LEAFLET MITRAL VALVE
7 LEFT ATRIUM
8 LEFT ATRIAL WALL

Using an echocardiogram to study the heart.

Why Are These Procedures Done?

An **ECG** is done for several reasons:
1. It may be done as a part of a routine physical after the age of 40.
2. It is also done to document the rate, rhythm, and general condition of the heart.
3. A third reason is to follow the course of a heart attack.
4. It is done to monitor heart rate and rhythm during surgery or other invasive procedures.

Holter and **telemetry monitoring** are done to document **dysrhythmias** (change in rhythm) during daily living activities. This is done over a specified length of time.

An **echocardiogram** is done to visualize the size, motion, and composition of the heart (wall motion, valve motion, accumulation of fluid, etc.) and great vessels as it is actually occurring.

A **vectorcardiogram** is done to see if the size and direction of the heart's electrical cur-

VECTORCARDIOGRAPHY

SAGITTAL HORIZONTAL FRONTAL

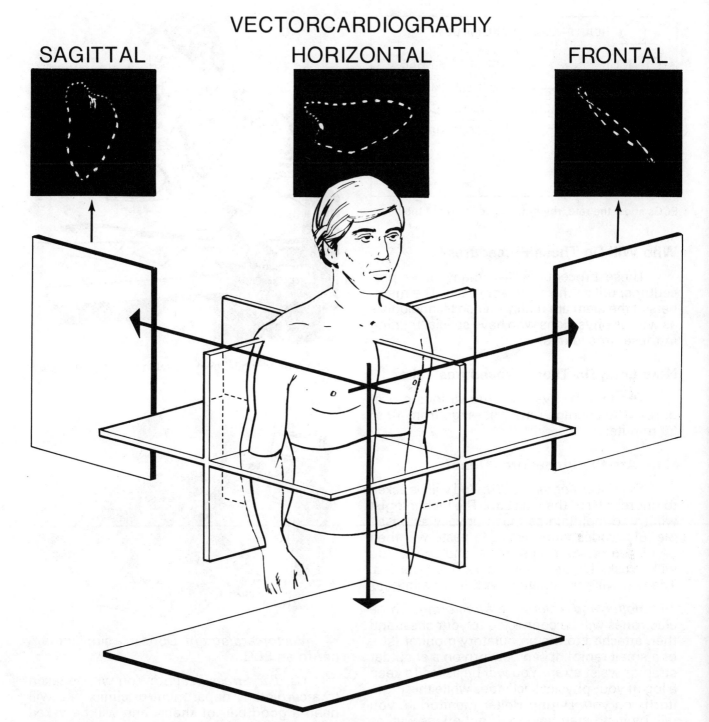

Vectorcardiograms show the direction and force of the heart's electrical activity.

rents are normal. This test aids in the diagnosis of muscular abnormalities.

 Cardiac stress testing is a *controlled* method of physically exerting the heart. The results of the physical exertion are graphically recorded by the electrocardiograph equipment.

 A **phonocardiogram** is a diagnostic procedure done to document the heart sounds in coordination with the ECG. It is a method of recording opening and closing of valves as well as extra heart sounds due to abnormalities.

Is There Any Preparation for These Procedures?

 No! These procedures, as was stated earlier, are non-invasive in nature. They may be done on an out-patient as well as an in-patient basis.

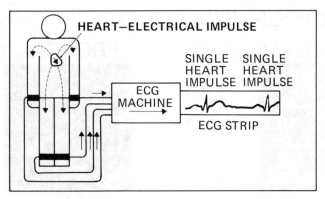

HEART—ELECTRICAL IMPULSE

SINGLE SINGLE
HEART HEART
IMPULSE IMPULSE

ECG MACHINE →

ECG STRIP

ECGs show the rate, rhythm, and condition of the heart.

Who Will Do These Procedures?

These procedures, like many other procedures, utilize the team approach. The members of the team are highly trained technologists as well as physicians who have special training in these procedures.

How Long Do These Procedures Take?

The time will vary for the various procedures. The average time will range from 10 to 30 minutes.

How Are the Procedures Done?

Electrocardiogram (ECG): You will be asked to undress from the waist up. The technologist will try to maintain as much privacy as possible. Electrodes with electrode paste will then be placed on your legs, arms, and chest. You will be asked to lie still as the ECG is recorded. The test will take only about 5 to 10 minutes.

Holter and Telemetry Monitoring: Three electrodes will be connected to your chest and then attached to the ambulatory monitor (size of a small radio). It can be worn on a shoulder strap or waist strap. You will be asked to keep a log of your physical activities while this monitor is on you. During Holter monitoring, you will be instructed how to turn it off, as well as where and when to return the unit.

Echocardiogram: You will be positioned on a table or bed and put into a hospital gown. The technologist will take care in maintaining as much privacy as possible. A gel, which is cool to the skin, will be placed on your skin over the heart region. A transducer will be moved over this area. A transducer is an electro-mechanical device used to convert one type of energy into another (sound waves to electrical signal). These signals are then recorded graphically or on photographic film.

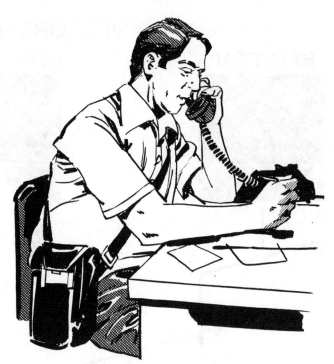

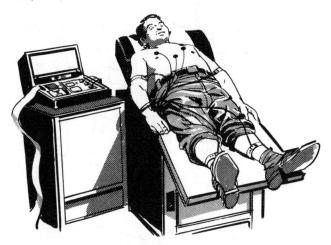

Holter monitoring (above) and telemetry monitoring (below).

Vectorcardiogram: Done in a similar manner to an ECG.

Cardiac Stress Testing: You will be taken to a cardiology department or clinic. You will need a good pair of shoes, and will be asked to put on a hosptial gown. At this time the technologist will connect you to an ECG monitor, and run a rhythm strip (a small sample of what your heart is doing at the start of the test). You will now be asked to step onto the treadmill. It is very similar to a conveyor belt. The physician will start the machine slowly and gradually work it up to a faster pace. During this time the physician will monitor your blood pressure and your ECG. The technologist will often ask you how you feel. At the end of the test the technologist will once again run a rhythm strip. A second method of doing a stress

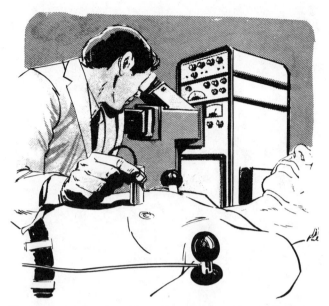

Technician using transducer to produce echocardiogram.

test is by having you ride a stationary (non-moving) bicycle. The same information is obtained.

Phonocardiogram: You will be taken to an ECG department or cardiology clinic for the procedure. There you will be placed on a table and asked to lie very still. The technologist will place a microphone on your chest and record the sounds. These microphones are moved from one area to another. The sounds recorded will depend on the placement of the microphone.

When Will I Know the Results?

As soon as the physician has all the data from the procedure, the results will be discussed with you and your family.

Are There Any Complications Or Side Effects?

The only cardiac non-invasive test that may lead to a complication is the cardiac stress test. The side effect that may occur is a **dysrhythmia** or a change in heart rhythm. Medications and emergency equipment are always available in the procedure area.

Will My Insurance Cover These Procedures?

Most insurance companies will cover the procedure and physician fee. The amount of coverage will differ from one insurance company to another.

Comments and Questions

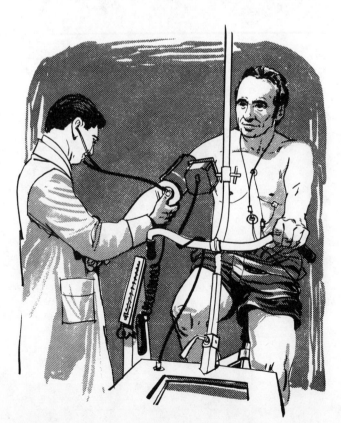

Stress testing to measure the heart's activity.

Your Guide to
Electrophysiology Studies

Introduction

Your doctor has requested that you have a special type of cardiac pacing study done. This study is called an electrophysiology study. It is important that you understand what this study is, why it is being done, and how it is done. In this information, you will find diagrams of the heart, a list of defined terms referring to the cardiac electrophysiology study, and a discussion of some of the most frequently asked questions concerning this procedure.

What Is a Cardiac Electrophysiology Study?

In defining this procedure let us take it word by word. *Cardiac* pertains to the heart. *Electro* pertains to electrical activity. *Physiology* pertains to a function of a body process. Combining these definitions, we come up with an electrical function of the heart. This is accomplished by insertion of a special pacing catheter and the results are recorded graphically on paper.

What Is the Heart's Electrical Function?

The electrical activity of the heart is controlled by the conduction system of the heart. The electrocardiogram (ECG) is the graphic picture of the electrical activity of the heart.

The conduction system of the heart is made up of a group of specialized cells. This system carries an electrical signal from its point of or-

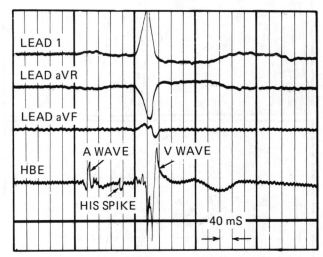

Example of an ECG tracing.

igin to the muscle fibers, resulting in the contraction of the heart, or heart beat. Below is a diagram of the heart's conduction system.
NOTE: There are six parts to the normal conduction system.

Why Is an Electrophysiology Study Done?

A cardiac electrophysiology study is done to determine if there is a cardiac electrical dysfunction and where the dysfunction is located.

What Are the Diagnostic Reasons for Having an Electrophysiology Study Done?

1. To evaluate the mechanism (re-entry, accessory pathway, ectopic foci, site (area), extent of **arrhythmia** (irregularity of rythm), and/or conduction defect.
2. To evaluate reasons for **syncope** (fainting). To look for a defect in impulse formation and/or conduction.
3. To evaluate drug or pacing therapy.

Is There Any Preparation for This Procedure?

Yes!
1. Food may be withheld until after the procedure.
2. You will be asked to put on a hospital gown the morning of the procedure.

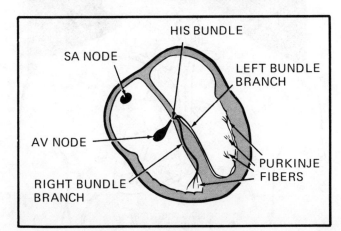

Electrical conduction system of the heart.

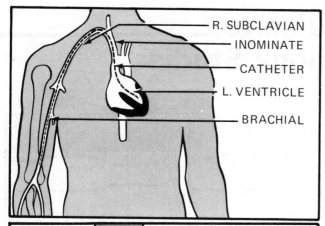

R. SUBCLAVIAN
INOMINATE
CATHETER
L. VENTRICLE
BRACHIAL

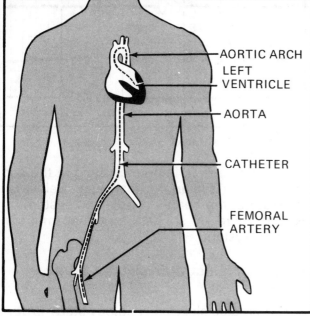

AORTIC ARCH
LEFT VENTRICLE
AORTA
CATHETER
FEMORAL ARTERY

Femoral artery approach for catheter placement.

3. The nurse will put a small needle into your vein for medication and/or fluids.
4. You will be given some medication prior to the test to help you relax. You will be in the lab for a while.

Where Is the Procedure Done?

This procedure may be done in an electrophysiology laboratory, cardiovascular laboratory, or X-ray special procedures.

Who Will Do the Procedure?

The cardiac electrophysiology procedure is done utilizing the team approach. The team members are highly trained technologists, nurses, and an invasive cardiologist. A **cardiologist** is a physician who specializes in disorders of the heart. The invasive cardiologist has special training in cardiac catheterization and electrophysiology procedures.

How Is the Procedure Done?

Electrophysiology procedures may be broken down into four distinct sections. These are: (1) the accurate measurement of waves and time intervals, (2) pacing studies (atrial, ventricular, sinus node, coronary sinus, His bundle, and atria and ventricle in combination), (3) drug challenge, and (4) mapping of the heart.

The general procedure discussed below is common to all these procedures.

You will be brought to the procedure room, assisted onto a table, and made as comfortable as possible. You will see a great deal of equipment in the room. A fluoroscopy machine (type of X-ray), a physiologic recorder (machine which records specific functions such as heart rate and His bundle wave forms, etc.), and ECG and defibrillator equipment to record and change the electrical activity of the heart, an instrument tray, and emergency equipment. Do not be frightened. All of this equipment is there for your safety and to make the test as meaningful as possible.

A member of the team will connect you to an ECG machine to monitor your heart rate and rhythm. This is done throughout the study. The physician will decide in which area to place the catheter (arm or leg). When this is done, a nurse or technologist and physician will clean

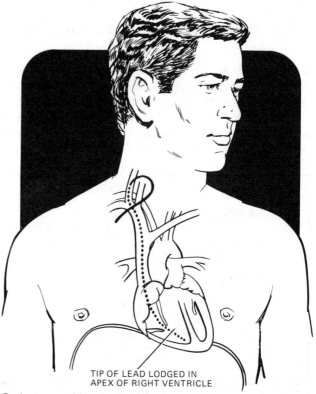

TIP OF LEAD LODGED IN APEX OF RIGHT VENTRICLE

Catheter position in the heart.

the area around which the catheter is to be inserted with an antiseptic (germ killing) solution. Establishment of a sterile (germ-free) field with sterile towels and sheets is the next step. It is very important that you *do not* touch this sterile field. The physician is now ready to inject the area with some numbing medication (anesthetic). (This is similar to what the dentist uses when working on your teeth.) It will sting; but it will only last for a few seconds. The doctor is now ready to insert the pacing catheter. This is done by first placing a needle in the vein, and then inserting the catheter through it. (This is known as the percutaneous approach.) You may feel some pressure, but you should not have any pain. There are *no* nerves in the blood vessels. The physician will now guide the catheter, with the aid of the fluoroscopy (X-ray) machine, into the area of the heart to be studied. The electrical signals from your heart are transmitted via the catheter and the ECG to the recorder, where they are put on paper. The physician, by use of a generator (batteries), may also stimulate your heart to beat faster. This is called **pacing study**. You may feel your heart beating faster. Do not be concerned about this. It is a normal feeling. The doctor may wish to give you some intravenous (through the vein) medication and record the results of it. This is called a **drug challenge**. The fourth section of the study mentioned was **mapping** of the heart. Done only in large hospitals, it is recording the rates of contraction of the individual muscle fibers. It is a long study, utilizing more than one catheter.

When the physician has obtained the information needed, the catheter is withdrawn, and pressure is held over the site until the bleeding stops. An antiseptic ointment is put over the puncture site, and a dry sterile dressing applied.

After the study, you will be taken back to your room to rest. Your heart rate and rhythm will continue to be monitored. The nurse will check you often. This is normal procedure.

When Will I Know the Results?

The physician will talk to you and your family after going over all the data.

Are There Any Complications or Side Effects?

As in any procedure there is always a slight chance of a complication occurring. However, the diagnostic benefit of having the procedure done far outweighs the risk. A few of the side effects that may occur are dysrhythmia (irregular rhythm), discomfort at insertion site, and infection, but these are rare.

Will My Insurance Cover This Procedure?

Most health insurance companies will cover the procedure and the physician fee. The amount of coverage will differ from one insurance company to another.

Terminology

Arrhythmia—change, abnormality of the cardiac rhythm.

Atria—the first chambers on either side of the heart that receive blood from veins.

Bradycardia—slow heart rate (less than 60 beats per minute).

Cardiac—pertaining to the heart.

Cardiovascular—pertaining to the heart and blood vessels.

Catheter—a hollow tube of hard or soft rubber.

Conduction—the passage or transfer of electrons.

Dysfunction (anatomic)—any abnormality in the function of an organ (e.g., heart)

Dysrhythmia—disordered rhythm

Ectopic focus—beat originating from an abnormal place.

Fluoroscopy—examination of internal body structures by X-ray.

Impulse—an electrical force or action usually of short duration.

Invasive—utilizing surgery, radiation, or intravenous/intra-arterial dyes.

Pacing—any substance or object that influences the rate at which a reaction occurs.

Percutaneous—performed through the skin.

Physiologic—pertaining to natural or normal processes.

Rhythm—action recurring at regular intervals.

Sinus rhythm—"normal" rhythm for the heart.

Syncope—fainting or swooning.

Tachycardia—fast heart rate (more than 100 beats per minute).

Ventricle—the lower chambers or second chambers on both sides of the heart that push the blood out of the heart into large arteries.

Comments and Questions

Your Guide to Pacemakers

Introduction

Your doctor has told you that you need a pacemaker. This information explains what a pacemaker is, how it works, and what it means to you and your family.

Your Heart and How It Works

The heart is a pump. It is a hollow organ, comprised of two walls that divide the heart into four chambers. The top two chambers are called **atria** and the bottom two chambers are called **ventricles**. The heart is made up of various layers of muscle. The heart has an area of special tissue that makes up the **conduction system**. The conduction system makes the heart contract or beat.

How Does the Conduction System Work?

The conduction system allows a signal to travel from its point of origin through a network of specialized cells throughout the heart. This results in a contraction or heart beat. This system is very similar to turning on a light switch, having the electricity flow through the wires, and then lighting the bulb.

This system is composed of six major divisions: (1) sino-atrial node (SA node, or pacemaker); (2) atrial pathways; (3) atrio-ventricular node (AV node); (4) bundle of His; (5) bundle branches; and (6) Purkinje system.

There are many reasons why a heart does not always beat regularly. For some reason,

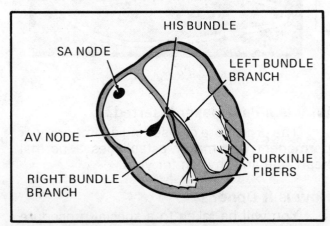

Electrical conduction system of the heart.

the signal that was started in the SA node does not travel all the way through the conduction system. It is blocked at one of the junctions or divisions of the conduction system. Remember the example of the lamp. This blockage is similar to a short or broken wire. You turn on the lamp switch, but the bulb does not light.

Due to this blockage, your heart rate may become very slow and irregular. This may be temporary or permanent. Some causes for these blockages are drugs, heart attack, trauma, and surgery.

What Is an Artificial Pacemaker?

An artificial pacemaker has two parts, a catheter (called a lead) and a generator. The lead has one or two electrodes at the end of it.

The lead is simply one or two wires covered by a plastic tube that carries the signal from its source (generator) to the heart. The electrodes on the end of the wire are the areas that come in direct contact with the heart muscle. This allows the signal to spread throughout the heart and causes the heart to beat or contract.

The generator is a special type of battery. It is the source of the signal.

What Is the Difference Between a Temporary and a Permanent Pacemaker?

A temporary pacemaker is just what it sounds like. It is inserted for a short time, usually three days to one week. The generator (battery) is on the outside of your body. It may be carried on a belt, in a pocket, or pinned to your gown or bed.

A permanent pacemaker is for full-time use. The generator is surgically inserted under your skin (internally).

Where Will the Procedure Be Done?

Pacemakers, temporary and permanent, may be done in several locations of the hospital: X-ray department, critical care units, special procedure areas, operating rooms, or emergency rooms. In extreme emergencies, the procedure may also be done at the patient's bedside.

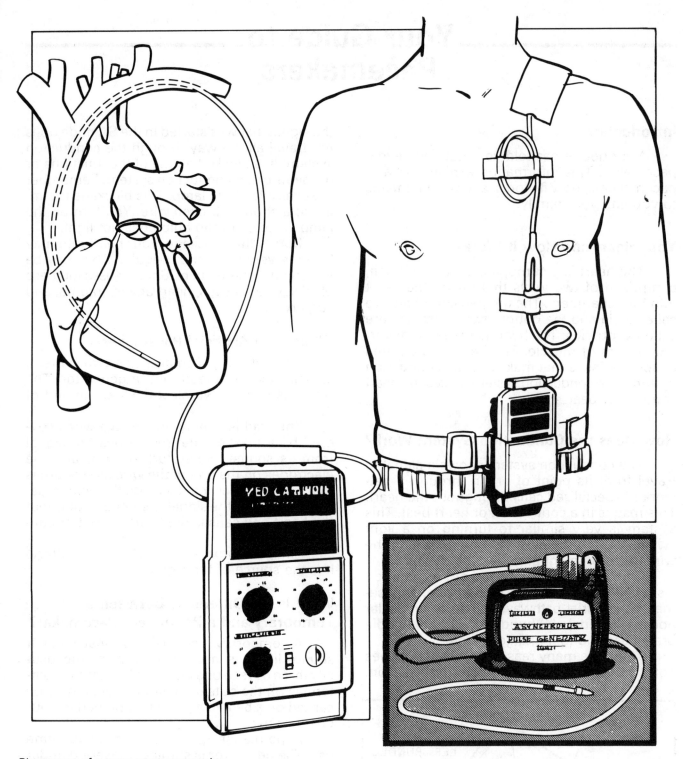

Placement of a temporary pacemaker.

When Will the Procedure Be Done?

Frequently, a temporary pacemaker will be done as an emergency procedure. This is usually due to a very low heart rate of 30 to 40 per minute, which has developed suddenly.

A permanent pacemaker *usually* is not an emergency procedure. It can be scheduled for a set date and time.

Why Is a Pacemaker Inserted?

The procedure of inserting a temporary or permanent pacemaker establishes a normal heart rate and rhythm for you.

How Is It Done?

You will be taken to a special procedure room where there will be trained personnel, an

X-ray machine called a fluoroscopy unit, an ECG monitor so the heart rate and rhythm can be constantly observed, and emergency equipment.

You will be moved onto an X-ray table and made as comfortable as possible.

A member of the team will connect you to an ECG machine so your heart rate and rhythm can be closely observed. A member of the team will frequently ask you how you feel. This is done because the staff wants you to be as comfortable as possible during the procedure.

At the beginning of the procedure, you will be requested to put your hands at your sides and *keep* them there. A team member will then clean the area where the pacemaker is to be inserted and establish a sterile (germ-free) field. This is done to help prevent an infection from occurring. Be sure you *do not* touch the sheets and towels! If you need to move, ask for some help.

The physician will then numb the area with an anesthetic. This is similar to the medicine the dentist uses to numb your mouth when he works on your teeth. After the area is numbed, the doctor will place a needle into a vein in your neck, chest, or usually your arm. Then the pacing lead will be inserted and positioned in the heart with the aid of the X-ray machine. During the entire procedure, team members will be watching your heart rate and rhythm closely. You may feel pressure from the doctor working, but you should feel no pain. There are *no* nerves inside the blood vessels. If this is a temporary pacemaker, the doctor will connect the ends of the lead to the external generator, and then check that it is working properly. If so, the lead will be sutured (sewn) in place. It will be covered with a dry sterile dressing. Then you will be returned to your room.

If, however, this is a permanent pacemaker, the physician will make a small incision, about 2½ inches in length, called a pocket, in the skin of your chest. This is the area where the generator will be placed, just under the skin.

The generator and lead will be tested to make sure they are functioning properly. Then the area will be sutured and dressed with a dry sterile dressing. You will now be returned to your room.

How Long Will It Take?

The average time is about 30 minutes for a temporary pacemaker and an hour for a permanent pacemaker. Everyone is a little different from everyone else, so your time may be longer or shorter.

Who Will Do the Procedure?

A doctor who is especially trained in this area. He or she may be a cardiologist or a surgeon.

What Happens After the Procedure?

When you return to your room, you will again be connected to an ECG monitor so your heart rate and rhythm can be monitored closely. You will be requested to stay in bed for 4 to 8 hours. This *does not* mean to get up and go to the bathroom. The nurses will be checking you frequently; if you need something for some minor discomfort, they will give it to you.

If you had a permanent pacemaker inserted, you may have a small drain that will come out in about 24 hours. You will also receive a temporary identification card. This card has the number of your pacemaker on it, and your doctor's name and address. You will be given a booklet of important facts about your new pacemaker.

Are There Any Complications or Side Effects?

As with any procedure, there is always a slight chance of a complication occurring. However, the benefit received from the procedure drastically outweighs not having the procedure done. The three main complications that may occur are irregular heart rhythm, infection, or pacemaker failure.

Does My Insurance Pay for This Procedure?

Most insurance companies will pay the majority of the hospital bill as well as the physician bill.

Comments and Questions

Your Guide to
Cardiac Catheterization

Introduction

Very soon you will undergo a diagnostic procedure or test known as cardiac catheterization. It is most important that you understand what this procedure is, and why it is being done.

Following are a list of defined terms concerning heart disease, and the answers to some of the most frequently asked questions about cardiac catheterization.

If, after reading this, you still have questions, feel free to ask your doctor or a member of the catheterization team. Write your questions down as you think of them. This way, you will be sure to remember them and the doctor will be able to answer them.

How Does Your Heart Work?

Your heart is a little larger than your fist. It weighs a little less than a pound. For such a small organ, it works very hard. Your heart is actually a pump. It pumps blood to the lungs and to the body.

Two walls, each called a **septum**, divide the heart into right and left, as well as up and down.

The septum divides the heart into four chambers or rooms. The upper ones are known as **atria** and the lower ones are known as **ventricles**. The septum also divides the heart into two sides, the right side and the left side.

Valves like one-way doors regulate the flow of the blood into and out of the heart. There are two valves on each side of the heart.

We have stated that the heart is a pump. It is really two pumps. The right side of the heart receives blood from the body. It is known as **venous** (dirty) blood because it is carrying a waste gas called **carbon dioxide**.

The heart pumps this blood to the lung where the carbon dioxide is exchanged for oxygen.

The oxygenated blood is then taken into the left side of the heart and pumped through the aorta to all parts of the body. The **aorta** is the largest artery in the body.

The heart, like every other organ in the body, must have a constant supply of oxygen and nutrients. It is also important that the waste material and gases are removed. This is done by the coronary circulation.

The two coronary arteries (right and left) are the first two branches from the aorta. They leave the aorta very close to the aortic valve of the heart.

Arteries and veins are like roads. These blood vessels allow the blood to travel to and from all parts of the body. However, if these "roads" become narrowed or blocked completely, it is difficult to get the correct amount of nutrients and oxygen to the tissue. It may even be impossible. When this happens in the heart, a signal is sent out that something is wrong. The signal is chest pain (**angina**). What happens if the artery is completely blocked? This means that NO nutrients or oxygen can get to that area of the heart. If that area of the heart has no collateral (back-up) blood supply (or side roads), then it dies. This is known as a **myocardial infarction** or heart attack.

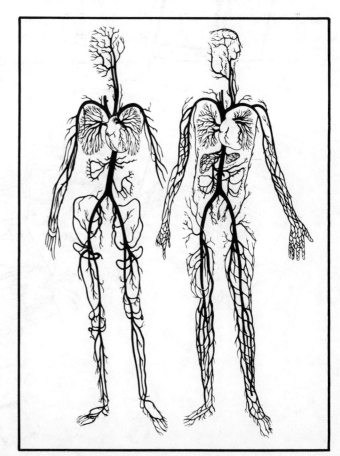

Circulation of the blood: arteries (left) and veins (right).

Who Receives Cardiac Catheterization?

1. People who have possible heart valve disease.
2. People who have questionable narrowing or blockage of the coronary vessels.
3. Children and young adults with congenital heart disease (disease present at birth).
4. People with heart disease of unknown etiology (cause).
5. People who have some form of trauma (injury) to the chest.

What Is Cardiac Catheterization?

Cardiac catheterization is a diagnostic test to study the chambers, valves, and the blood supply to the heart and the body.

Why Is Cardiac Catheterization Done?

1. To determine the cause of chest pain.
2. To locate the damage and the extent of the damage after a heart attack.
3. To establish the suitability of a patient for open heart surgery.
4. To determine the function of the heart after heart surgery.
5. Other reasons for which it may be done:
   a. Valve disease
   b. Arrhythmias (abnormal heart beat patterns)
   c. Hypertension (high blood pressure)
   d. Congenital heart disease (birth disease or defect)
   e. Chest trauma
   f. Congestive heart failure
   g. Myopathy (abnormal heart muscle function)
   h. Diagnosed coronary disease (partial blockages in the coronary arteries)

Where Is Cardiac Catheterization Done?

1. Location of cardiac catheterization laboratories:
   a. X-ray

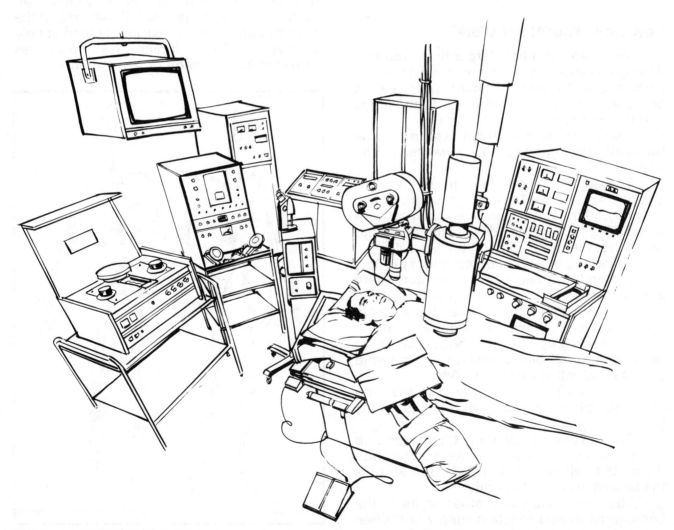

Cardiac catheterization laboratory.

b. Surgery
c. Cardiac clinics
d. Special area defined for cardiac catheterization
2. Several hospitals are able to do this study. The choice of the hospital is a decision that you and your physician will make.

How Is a Cardiac Catheterization Done?

1. Cardiac catheterization may be done by either of two methods.
   a. **Femoral Approach**—The groin area is prepped and numbed with a local anesthetic (like the dentist uses). A catheter is then introduced into an artery or vein and moved to the heart. The doctor watches the catheter as it advances into the heart. A special X-ray machine (fluoroscope) lets the doctor see the catheter. Once the catheter is in the blood vessel, you will feel no discomfort. There are no nerves in the blood vessels. The physician will record pressures, and will inject some dye to look at the blood vessels and the main pumping chamber of the heart. When dye is injected into the ventricle (pump), you feel warm all over. It is a normal response and lasts only a few seconds. You will not experience this feeling when the coronaries are injected because so little dye is used. At the end of the study, the catheter is removed. Pressure is held over the area where the catheter was put in until the bleeding has stopped. A dressing will be put over the site, and you will be returned to your room.
   b. **Brachial Approach**—This is very similar to the femoral approach except that the arm is used. In this method, a small incision is made to introduce the catheter into the blood vessel. The rest of the procedure is the same as the femoral approach.

Other Frequently Asked Questions

1. *What does the room look like?*
   When entering the cardiac catheterization lab, you will see a great deal of equipment. There will be an X-ray machine with a camera and TV monitors to view the inside of the heart. There will also be an ECG monitor and a table with instruments on it.
2. *Will there be much pain?*
   No! You will be given some medication before you come to the lab to help you relax. Once you are in the lab, you will be given a local anesthetic in the area where the catheter will be placed to make the area numb.
3. *Why can't I be put to sleep?*
   We need your help! You will be asked to take very deep breaths, and may be asked to cough at times.
4. *Why are the deep breaths necessary?*
   There is a muscle called the **diaphragm** that partially covers the heart. When a deep breath is taken, the diaphragm moves down in the abdomen. This exposes that part of the heart.
5. *How long does catheterization take?*
   The average length of time is about an hour. More than half of this time is spent in getting you ready for the test and in clean-up time after the test. The catheter is only in your heart about 10 to 15 minutes.
6. *What is the difference between having the test done through the leg or the arm?*
   Both methods are used. However, about 90% of the procedures are done through the leg. There is no need for an incision in the leg. A small incision is needed for the arm because the blood vessels are smaller.
7. *What are the complications?*
   As in any type of diagnostic test, there is always a slight chance of complications occurring. These include chest discomfort and temporary palpitations. Rarely (2 in 10,000), ventricular fibrillation (fast, irregular heart beat) occurs. This needs electrical shock to recover. More rarely still, is a heart attack or sudden death (2 in 100,000). These complications occur more frequently in the extremely ill patient.
8. *When will I know the results?*
   Your doctor will talk to you about the results the next day. A great deal of information has to be reviewed and pictures studied before the results are known.
9. *Will my insurance cover the procedure?*
   Cardiac catheterization is an expensive procedure. It requires highly trained personnel and expensive equipment. Most insurance companies will pay for the procedure and also for the professional fees of the physicians.

Terminology

Aneurysm—localized dilation (weakening) of the blood vessel wall.

Angina—constricting or pressure-type of chest pain due to lack of oxygen to the heart muscle.

Artery—the blood vessels that carry oxygenated blood from the heart to the body.

Bypass graft—the "tying in" of a new, patent (open) blood vessel around an occluded (blocked) one.

Cardiac, cardium, cardial—heart.

Congenital heart disease—heart disease that has existed since birth.

Congestive heart failure—a condition resulting when the heart is no longer able to contract forcefully enough to propel blood out to all parts of the body.

Coronary Occlusion—blockage of coronary artery.

Embolus—a plug or clot that moves from its point of origin.

Heart—a muscular organ that, by contracting, pushes blood to the lungs and to all parts of the body.

Hypertension—high blood pressure.

Infarct—death of tissue.

Myocardial infarct—death of a section of the heart muscle.

Insufficiency—a valve that leaks.

Myo—muscle.

Myocardium—heart muscle.

Open heart surgery—direct surgical repair of the heart by means of an incision through the chest wall.

Premature beats—extra beats, sometimes referred to by patients as palpitations.

Thrombus—a plug or clot in a blood vessel or one of the cavities of the heart, which remains at the point of its formation.

Stenosis—a narrowing or constriction.

Valve—a door that lets the blood flow in only one direction.

Veins—the blood vessels through which blood is returned to the heart from the body.

Comments and Questions

Your Guide to Pericardiocentesis

Introduction

Your doctor has ordered a special examination for you called pericardiocentesis. This test may also be referred to as cardiocentesis. In this information, many of the questions you may have concerning the procedure will be discussed.

What Is Pericardiocentesis?

Pericardiocentesis is the aspiration (withdrawal) of fluid from the pericardial space (space around the heart) to relieve pressure on the heart. This fluid is then sent to the laboratory for diagnostic testing.

Why Is Pericardiocentesis Done?

Pericardiocentesis is done for one of two reasons. To relieve pressure exerted on the heart by the buildup of fluid around the heart, or to obtain a sample of the fluid for diagnostic purposes. The buildup of fluid may be due to trauma, infections, tumors, pericarditis, etc.

Is There Any Special Preparation?

Yes!
1. You will be asked to put on a hospital gown.
2. Food may be withheld until after the procedure.
3. A small needle will be inserted in the vein for fluids and/or medications, if you do not already have one.
4. You may be given some medication before the test to help you relax.

Where Will the Procedure Be Done?

The procedure will be done in a special procedure area or in a critical care unit. In emergency situations, the procedure may be done in the emergency room, operating room, cardiac catheterization laboratory, or X-ray department. Although not essential, a fluoroscopy unit (type of X-ray) is very helpful during this procedure.

Who Will Do the Procedure?

This procedure, like many others, utilizes a team approach. The team is made up of nurse, technologists (X-ray, ECG), and a physician. All the members of the team have had special training in this procedure.

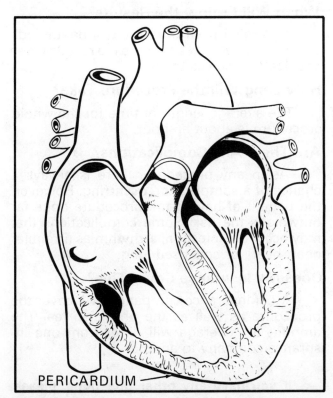

PERICARDIUM

Diagram of the heart showing the pericardium.

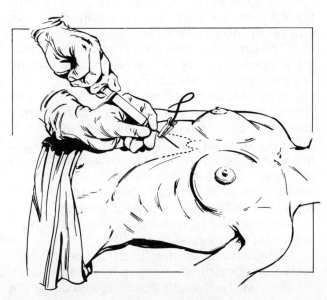

Area of needle insertion for pericardiocentesis.

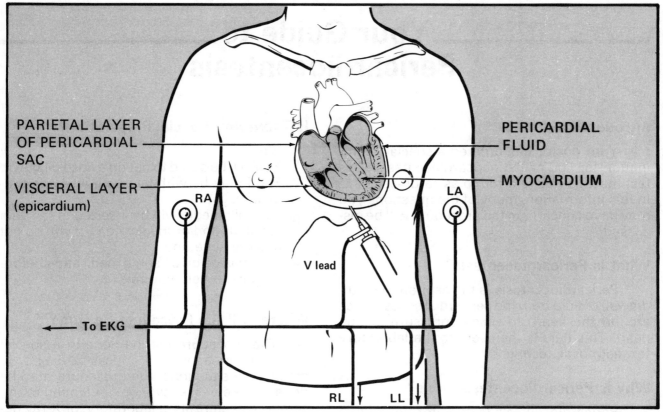

PARIETAL LAYER
OF PERICARDIAL
SAC

VISCERAL LAYER
(epicardium)

RA

V lead

To EKG

PERICARDIAL
FLUID

MYOCARDIUM

LA

RL   LL

Diagram of pericardiocentesis procedure.

How Is the Procedure Done?

You will be placed on an X-ray table or bed in a semirecumbent position (head will be elevated 30 to 60 degrees). A member of the medical team will connect you to an ECG (electrocardiograph) monitor. Your heart rate and rhythm will be watched carefully during the entire procedure.

At this point, the area of the chest to be entered will be washed with an antiseptic solution (germ killer), and sterile (germ-free) sheets placed over the area. It is very important that you *do not* touch these sheets.

The physician will now inject some numbing medication, like the dentist uses, around the area to be entered. This may sting but it will only last a short time. The doctor is now ready to insert the needle. You will feel pressure, but should feel no pain. The needle is guided into place by fluoroscopy and the ECG monitor. When the doctor has reached the correct area, the fluid will be withdrawn slowly with a syringe or perhaps a vacuum bottle, and then sent to the laboratory for analysis.

As the fluid is withdrawn, you may find it is a great deal easier to breathe.

When most of the fluid has been withdrawn, the doctor will remove the needle, clean the area with antiseptic solution, and cover the site with a bandaid.

When you return to your room, the nurses will check you often. They will check your vital signs (blood pressure, pulse, respiration), and the site where you had your test done.

When Will I Know the Results?

The relief from pressure will be immediate. You will be told about the lab results when the doctor receives them.

How Long Will the Procedure Take?

The average length of time for the whole procedure is about an hour.

Are There Any Complications?

As in any procedure, there is always a chance of a complication occurring. However, the benefit of having the procedure done far outweighs the risk. Some complications that may occur are infection, arrhythmias (irregular heart beat), or collapsed lung.

Does My Insurance Cover This?

Most insurance companies will cover the procedure as well as the physician fee. The amount of coverage will differ from one insurance company to another.

If you have any other questions, please contact your doctor.

Your Guide to Elective Cardioversion

Introduction

Your doctor has ordered a special examination for you called an elective cardioversion. This information discusses many of your questions concerning the test.

What Is an Elective Cardioversion?

An **elective cardioversion** is a method to terminate **tachydysrhythmias** (fast, irregular heart rhythms) by use of a synchronized (timed) direct current charge.

Why Is an Elective Cardioversion Done?

An elective cardioversion is done to re-establish a normal heart rate and rhythm for you.

Is There Any Preparation for the Test?

Yes!
1. Food may be withheld until after the test.
2. If you have dentures, you will be asked to remove them.
3. A small needle will be inserted for the administration of medication.
4. You will be asked to put on a hospital gown.

Where Is the Procedure Done?

Elective cardioversion may be done in any one of a number of places in the hospital setting. Some of these areas may be the coronary care unit, emergency room, cardiology clinic

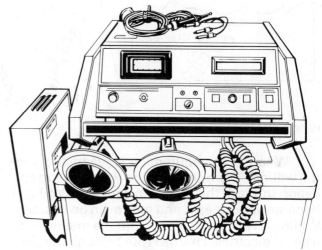

Equipment used for cardioversion.

or department, cardiac catheterization laboratory, special procedure unit, or even at the patient's bedside.

Who Will Do the Procedure?

This procedure, like many other procedures, is a team effort. There will be a nurse and a physician present and perhaps an ECG (Electrocardiographic) technician. All on the team are trained in the cardioversion procedure.

How Is the Procedure Done?

You will be taken to the area where the procedure is to be done and made as comfortable as possible on a table or bed. A member of the medical team will expose your chest and connect you to an ECG monitor. Your heart rate and rhythm are watched carefully throughout the procedure.

The needle in your arm will be tested to make sure that it is working properly.

A gelatin (jelly-like substance) is spread on two paddles. (Some hospitals use a cream, saline pads, or defib pads [jelly-like pads] instead of the gelatin.) This gelatin is cold to the skin. One of the paddles, called a posterior paddle, is placed under your back. (The physician will check the ECG pattern, and the cardioverter equipment.) The other paddle, called an anterior paddle, will be placed on your chest.

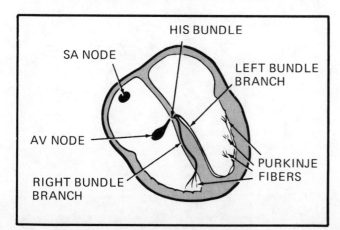

Electrical conduction system of the heart.

HIS BUNDLE

SA NODE

LEFT BUNDLE BRANCH

AV NODE

PURKINJE FIBERS

RIGHT BUNDLE BRANCH

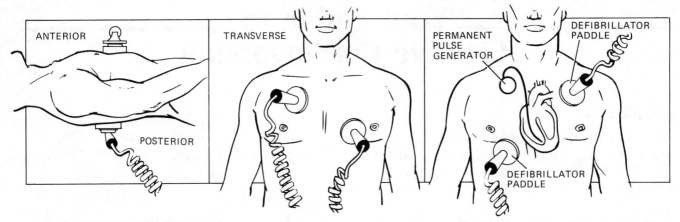

Paddle placement for cardioversion.

When all the equipment is ready, the doctor will ask the nurse to give you some medication through the needle in your arm. You will become very sleepy, and may even go to sleep. While you are very sleepy from the medication, a small electrical charge is put through the paddles. This charge allows the entire heart muscle to contract, thereby enabling the heart to resume a regular rate and rhythm. Some patients feel mild discomfort, but most of the patients do not remember the test at all!

When the cardioversion is over, you will be taken back to your room. Your heart rate and rhythm will be watched carefully for the next several hours. You will probably sleep for a period of time from the medication.

How Long Does the Procedure Take?

The actual cardioversion only takes a few seconds. The whole procedure takes about 10 to 15 minutes.

When Will I Know the Results?

The results are immediate, and your physician will tell you right after the procedure.

Are There Any Complications?

As in any procedure, there is always a small chance of a complication occurring. However, the benefit derived from the procedure far outweighs not having it done! Most common side effects are mild discomfort, temporary redness where the paddles were, and an irregular heart rhythm.

Will My Insurance Cover the Procedure?

Most insurance companies will cover the procedure as well as the physician fee. The amount will differ from one company to another.

Comments and Questions

4
Pulmonary Procedures

Sputum Collection

Sputum collection and laboratory analysis is an important diagnostic aid in the management of the patient with acute or chronic lung disease.

The main purpose of a sputum collection is to identify and/or isolate cells, fungus, bacteria, etc., as a primary cause for lung disease. Some diseases that may be diagnosed in this manner are bronchitis, pneumonia, abscesses, tuberculosis, and occasionally cancer.

Nurse's Responsibilities

Pre-Test
1. The most important aspect of a sputum collection is to ensure that it is collected correctly. Thus the explanation given to the patient must be clear, concise, and easily understood. The normal method of collecting such a specimen is the expectoration of sputum raised from the lungs and placed into a special container.
2. Explain how to use the sputum container and the importance of coughing deeply.
3. Best collected early in the morning on first arising.
4. If patient is receiving pulmonary treatments (IPPB or aerosol), may have better results in collecting.

Precautions
1. Have patient cough from deep in chest in order *not* to obtain an upper respiratory specimen.
2. Explain to the patient the importance of not contaminating the sputum cup.

Post-Procedure
   Send specimen to laboratory.

Pulmonary Function Tests

Pulmonary function tests are studies done to evaluate the ventilatory function of patients with suspected or confirmed pulmonary dysfunction. These studies are usually done in a pulmonary function laboratory by respiratory technologists. These studies may include tidal volume, minute volume, inspiratory and expiratory reserve volume, residual volume, vital and inspiratory functional residual and total lung capacity, among others.

The purposes of these studies are: (1) to determine the etiology of dyspnea; (2) to evaluate disability for insurance and/or legal purposes; (3) to determine the extent of lung disease; (4) to assess drug or other therapeutic regimens; and (5) to assess whether a pulmonary problem is restrictive or obstructive.

Nurse's Responsibilities:

Pre-Test
1. Explain the tests to the patient, and that they may be done on an out-patient basis.
2. Instruct the patient not to smoke 4 to 6 hours prior to the tests.
3. Encourage the patient to eat a small meal prior to the tests.
4. All medications with a sedative action should be withheld until after the tests.
5. Have the patient void prior to the tests.
6. Explain that these tests will take a lot of co-operation on his or her part.

Precautions
1. Patient must be able to cooperate.
2. Gastric extension due to a large meal will interfere with pulmonary tests.
3. Sedative drugs will decrease inspiratory and expiratory force.
4. Pregnancy may cause displacement of lung volume.
5. Loose or absent teeth may cause a leak around the mouth piece.

Post-Procedure
1. Allow patient to rest!
2. Order a snack or late tray if patient missed a meal.
3. Resume all previous orders.

Chest Physiotherapy

Chest physiotherapy is a mechanical means used to loosen secretions from the chest. It is also done to aid in the drainage of these secretions to higher respiratory levels through postural drainage. The latter effects easier removal of the secretions.

The purpose of these procedures is to loosen and drain congested lung areas due to thick mucous secretions. Patients who benefit from such procedures are those who have cystic fibrosis, pneumonia, bronchitis, and other lung diseases.

These procedures may be done in the patient's room or in respiratory or physical therapy departments.

Nurse's Responsibilities

Pre-Test
1. Explain the procedure to the patient (may be done as an out-patient).
2. Food is withheld until after the procedure, or the physiotherapy is scheduled between meals.
3. The physiotherapy should be scheduled in such a way as to leave adequate rest periods for the patient.
4. Family members should be encouraged to learn the techniques if this is a chronic condition.
5. Make available an adequate supply of pillows and tissues.

Precautions
1. Patient should be cooperative.
2. Patient should have adequate time to rest before and after procedure. Being tired will interfere with the test.
3. Physiotherapy should not be scheduled immediately after eating.

Post-Procedure
1. Allow patient to rest.
2. Provide the patient with tissues and/or sputum containers.
3. Order late meal tray if necessary.
4. Encourage fluid intake.

Chest X-Ray

A chest X-ray is the most common radiograph done. When a chest X-ray is ordered on a patient with a pulmonary problem, the physician is looking for signs of an infiltrate, fluids, tumor, foreign bodies, or other abnormalities. They are seen very clearly on the film because the lungs (pulmonary tissue) are radiolucent.

Nurse's Responsibilities

Pre-Test
1. Explain procedure to the patient (may be done as an out-patient).
2. Have patient put on a hospital gown and remove jewelry.
3. Assist patient in getting ready for transfer to radiology department. (X-ray may be done in patient's room if necessary.)

Precautions
1. Ask all female patients if they may be pregnant.
2. If patient is in critical care with multiple tubes, check to see that none has been dislodged during positioning.

3. Leave immediate area while patient is being radiographed to avoid unnecessary exposure.

Post-Procedure
None

Bronchoscopy

Bronchoscopy is the direct visualization of the tracheobronchial tree by means of a bronchoscope. A flexible fiberoptic bronchoscope is used frequently because of less trauma due to its size.

Bronchoscopy is done for two reasons: (1) as a diagnostic procedure; and (2) as a therapeutic procedure. Diagnostically, the procedure may be done (1) to visually examine the tracheobronchial tree for tumor, foreign bodies, bleeding site; and (2) to assist in the diagnosis of infections, tumors, etc., through obtaining sputum samples and biopsies for laboratory analysis. Therapeutically, the bronchoscopy may be done to remove foreign bodies, mucous plugs, or other obstructions from the tracheobronchial tree.

Nurse's Responsibilities

Pre-Test
1. Explain the procedure to the patient and family. (May be done as out-patient, but usually done on in-patients.)
2. Check to see that a permit has been signed. If not, have one signed and witnessed.
3. Check chart for allergic history to anesthetics, contrast media, etc.
4. Patient will be NPO for 6 to 12 hours prior to the study.
5. Ensure that there are recent X-ray and laboratory data available.
6. Instruct patient to remove dentures prior to procedure.
7. Have patient put on a hospital gown.
8. Have patient void prior to procedure.
9. Inform patient that he or she will be given medication to help relax during procedure.
10. Check IV for signs of infiltration. If patient does not have one, start one with an 18g or larger needle.
11. Inform the patient that the spray they will use to numb the throat does not taste good. It is used to suppress the gag reflex.
12. Get the patient and chart ready for transfer.
13. On call for the procedure, give pre-medication as per order.

Precautions
1. If examination is done while patient is awake, he or she should be cooperative, able to understand, and follow orders.
2. If samples of tissue or sputum are taken, label correctly and send to laboratory.
3. If procedure is done on an emergency basis, be prepared for possible aspiration due to vomiting. (Patient may have eaten very recently.)

4. The procedure is contraindicated in patients with respiratory failure.
5. Keep a tracheotomy tray at bedside for 24 hours.

Post-Procedure
1. Position unconscious patient on his side with head slightly elevated to prevent aspiration.
2. Position conscious patient in a semi-Fowler's position.
3. Monitor vital signs as per order.
4. Do not allow the patient to eat or drink until the gag reflex is present.
5. Supply patient with tissues and an emesis basin to expectorate saliva rather than swallowing it.
6. Inform physician immediately if any of these symptoms are present: (1) respiratory distress; (2) bleeding; or (3) subcutaneous crepitus.
7. Inform patient to refrain from coughing if he has had a biopsy taken. ("May dislodge the clot at the biopsy site.")
8. Instruct the patient *not* to smoke for several hours post-procedure.
9. Give analgesics as per order.
10. Inform the patient and family that hoarseness, sore throat, and loss of voice are common after this procedure and are only *temporary*.

Bronchography

Bronchography is a radiographic procedure utilizing contrast media to outline the tracheobronchial tree. It is not utilized as often today due to the advent of tomography, CAT scan, and the fiberoptic flexible bronchoscopes.

Bronchography may be done concurrently with a bronchoscopy. This procedure provides the physician with a permanent record of a pathologic process. It may also be done to guide the physician to a specific area in the lung while performing a bronchoscopy.

Nurse's Responsibilities

Pre-Test
See Bronchoscopy.

Precautions
1. Bronchography, like other radiographs, are contraindicated in pregnancy.
2. If patient is allergic to iodine, the procedure may be done if he or she is first prepped with steroids.
3. This procedure, like the bronchoscopy, is contraindicated in patients with severe respiratory failure.
4. Be alert for signs and symptoms of airway occlusion, laryngeal spasm, or other respiratory problems.
5. A tracheotomy tray should be at bedside for 24 hours.
6. The area should be equipped with emergency medications and equipment.

Post-Procedure
See Bronchoscopy.

Thoracentesis

Thoracentesis is a procedure where the thoracic wall is percutaneously punctured with a needle. This procedure is done diagnostically to obtain a pleural fluid sample for analysis, and therapeutically to relieve respiratory distress due to compression or hypoxemia by withdrawing pleural fluid, or to instill therapeutic agents directly into the pleural space.

Nurse's Responsibilities

Pre-Test
1. Explain procedure to patient and family.
2. Check chart to see if a permit has been signed. If not, have one signed and witnessed.
3. Food may be withheld until after the procedure, but not in every case.
4. Check IV for infiltration. If patient does not have an IV, start one with an 18g or larger needle.
5. Have patient put on a hospital gown.
6. Ask patient and check chart for past medical history of allergies and/or bleeding tendencies.
7. Inform that patients will be asked to hold their breath.
8. Inform the patient that the physician may use ultrasound or X-ray to help locate the correct area.
9. Instruct the patient not to make any sudden moves. This will minimize the risk of internal injuries.
10. Give pre-medication as per order.

Precautions
1. Patient should be able to cooperate.
2. This procedure would be contraindicated in patients with a bleeding disorder.
3. Be alert for signs and symptoms of respiratory distress (pneumo- or tension pneumothorax, mediastinal shift) or bleeding.
4. Correctly label and send all specimens to laboratory for analysis.
5. If patient is taking an antibiotic, relay this information on to the laboratory.

Post-Procedure
1. Position the patient on the affected side for 1 to 2 hours to help seal the puncture site. Elevate head to facilitate breathing.
2. Monitor vital signs as per order.
3. If post-procedure radiography has been ordered, help position the patient.
4. Observe the puncture site for drainage.
5. Observe patient for signs and symptoms of respiratory distress, cardiac problems due to mediastinal shift, reaccumulation of pleural effusion, pulmonary edema, and bleeding. Report any of these problems immediately to the physician.

Needle Biopsy of the Lung

A needle biopsy of the lung is usually accomplished via a transthoracic percutaneous approach. It is done to aid in the diagnosis of pleural effusions, pneumonia, pleural diseases, cancer, fungal diseases, etc.

Nurse's Responsibilities

Pre-Test
See Thoracentesis.

Precautions
See Thoracentesis.

Post-Procedure
See Thoracentesis.

Closed Thoracostomy By Means of a Chest Tube

A closed thoracostomy is often done as an emergency procedure. Listed below are some of the indications for this procedure: (1) to remove solids from the pleural space (chest trauma). These would include fibrin and blood clots. (2) To remove liquids from the pleural space, hemothorax (blood), aspirations (gastric and/or chemical), empyema (pus), pleural effusions (serous, blood, etc.); (3) to remove gases from the pleural space (air); and (4) to reexpand a collapsed lung by restoring negative pressure to the pleural space.

The insertion of a chest tube is done by the percutaneous transthoracic approach. The position of the tube or tubes will depend on the pathologic process. They are usually placed basilar and/or apical. (Inserted to withdraw blood and air from pleural cavity.) The chest tube is then connected to an underwater seal (closed chest) drainage.

Nurse's Responsibilities

Pre-Test
1. Explain the procedure to the patient and family.
2. If this is an emergency procedure, a family member may sign the permit.
3. Check IV for infiltration. If the patient does not have an IV, start one with an 18g or larger needle.
4. Assist the physician in positioning the patient if the procedure is to be done at the bedside.
5. Check the chart for any past history of allergies to anesthetics or bleeding problems.
6. Have the patient put on a hospital gown.
7. Keep patient NPO until after the procedure.
8. Instruct the patient that it is very important that he or she cooperates and does not move.
9. Give pre-medication as per order.
10. Emergency equipment and medications should be readily available.

Precautions
1. Have several clamps in room to use in clamping the chest tube if needed.
2. Always keep chest drainage containers below the height of the chest.
3. Milk tubes often to clear clots that may obstruct the drainage tube.
4. Take care that chest tubes are not pulled out or dislodged in positioning patient.
5. If any signs of breakage or leaking in the closed system occur, tighten all connections, listen for air leaks, clamp chest tubes, and notify physician.

Post-Procedure
1. Position patient as per physician order with head of bed slightly elevated to facilitate breathing.
2. Vital signs are to be monitored as per order.
3. Observe the type and amount of chest drainage.
4. Assist the patient in turning. Inform the patient it is very important that the tubes are not dislodged.
5. Milk or strip the chest tubes often to prevent clots from occurring.
6. Instruct the patient that he or she is *not* to get out of bed without help.
7. Clamp the chest tubes if you have to transport the patient.
8. Keep clamps and sterile dressings at the bedside for emergency use.
9. Check insertion site for drainage and/or signs of infection.
10. Always clamp tubes when changing drainage system.
11. Medicate with analgesics as per order.

Your Guide to Sputum Collection

Introduction

Your doctor has ordered a laboratory analysis of your sputum. This information will discuss the methods of obtaining the sample, why it is important, and other areas of interest.

What Is a Sputum Collection?

A **sputum collection** is a sample of mucous secretions from your respiratory tract.

Why Is a Sputum Collection Done?

A sputum collection is done to aid in the diagnosis of acute and chronic lung diseases. This is accomplished by having the mucous secretions tested in the laboratory for cellular content and/or for germ content. These two laboratory areas are called **cytology** (study of cells) and **bacteriology** (study of bacteria). Other special laboratory tests may be ordered on the same mucus specimen.

Is There Any Special Preparation For Collecting This Specimen?

Yes! It will be necessary that you obtain a sterile (germ-free) specimen container from the doctor or hospital. This test may be done on an out-patient basis.

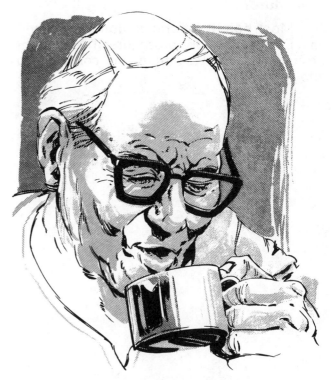
Coughing into cup for sputum specimen.

How Do You Collect This Specimen?

It is very important that the sputum be collected properly. Otherwise, the laboratory data may not show what is the real problem. When you remove the top from the container, be careful not to touch the inside of it. Lay the cover upside down with the outer surface closest to the table. Now it is important that you cough *very deeply from your chest* and expectorate (spit) the mucus into the container. Be careful not to touch the inside of the container. Pick up the lid by the rim and replace the lid on the container. It may take more than a single time to get the specimen. Follow the same procedure each time. If you do not cough deeply from the chest, the mucus will just be from the upper airway passages. This specimen will not give the doctor the necessary information.

When you have collected the specimen, give it to the nurse or if you are at home, take it to the place your doctor asked you to take it (office or hospital laboratory).

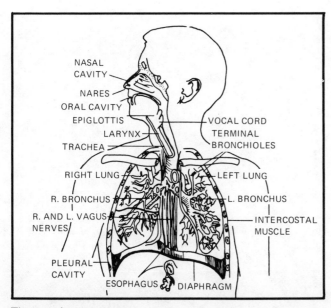

The respiratory system.

NASAL CAVITY
NARES
ORAL CAVITY
EPIGLOTTIS
LARYNX
TRACHEA
RIGHT LUNG
R. BRONCHUS
R. AND L. VAGUS NERVES
PLEURAL CAVITY
ESOPHAGUS
DIAPHRAGM
VOCAL CORD
TERMINAL BRONCHIOLES
LEFT LUNG
L. BRONCHUS
INTERCOSTAL MUSCLE

When Will I Know the Results?

The doctor will talk to you and your family when the laboratory report is received.

Will My Insurance Cover This Laboratory Procedure?

Most health insurance companies will cover this laboratory procedure. The amount of coverage will vary from one company to another.

Comments and Questions

Your Guide to Pulmonary Function Testing

Introduction

Your doctor has requested that you have a special lung test done. It is called pulmonary function testing. In this information, you will find a discussion of some of the most frequently asked questions concerning this procedure.

What Is Pulmonary Function?

Pulmonary function refers to the role of the bronchopulmonary system (major respiratory passages and lungs) in respiratory gas exchange of oxygen (O_2) and carbon dioxide (CO_2).

What Is Pulmonary Function Testing?

Pulmonary function testing is the clinical study of the lungs, which includes: (1) capacity, load, and stress tests; and (2) physiologic measurements.

Why Are Pulmonary Function Tests Done?

Pulmonary function tests are done to determine the nature of pulmonary dysfunction, and to what extent the lungs are damaged.

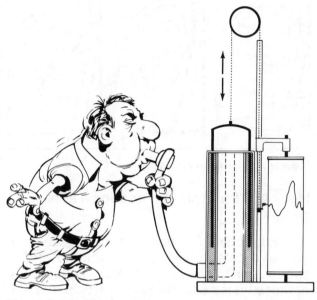
Measuring lung volume.

Is There Any Preparation for the Test?

Yes!
1. These tests may be done on an out-patient as well as in-patient basis.
2. Do not smoke for 4 to 6 hours prior to the test.
3. A large meal prior to the test may cause gastric distention, which may interfere with pulmonary function by restriction.

Where Are Pulmonary Function Studies Done?

Pulmonary function studies are done in a pulmonary laboratory. The pulmonary laboratory is usually located in the respiratory therapy department.

Who Will Do the Pulmonary Function Test?

The pulmonary function tests are done by highly trained pulmonary technologists. The data from the tests is reported by a physician who specializes in pulmonary problems.

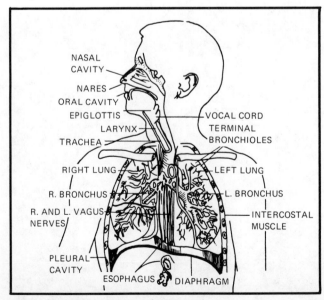

NASAL CAVITY
NARES
ORAL CAVITY
EPIGLOTTIS
LARYNX
TRACHEA
VOCAL CORD
TERMINAL BRONCHIOLES
RIGHT LUNG
LEFT LUNG
R. BRONCHUS
L. BRONCHUS
R. AND L. VAGUS NERVES
INTERCOSTAL MUSCLE
PLEURAL CAVITY
ESOPHAGUS
DIAPHRAGM

The respiratory system.

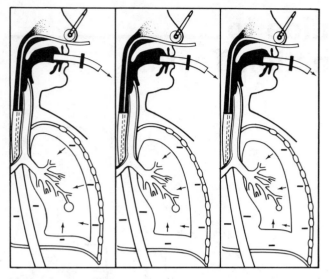

Measuring ventilatory capacity.

How Are Pulmonary Function Tests Done?

Pulmonary function tests are broken down into two categories: (1) lung volume and its subdivisions; and (2) ventilatory capacity. All of these tests need the active participation and cooperation of you, the patient. There are several parts to the tests. They all involve breathing into different pieces of equipment. The technologist will guide you through each phase of the tests. None of the tests is uncomfortable or painful! You may find that you are tired or out of breath after a few of the tests. A blood sample may be drawn to determine the levels of pH (acidity or alkalinity of the blood), O_2, and CO_2 in the blood. This provides data about the cardiopulmonary (heart-lung) function.

When Will I Know the Results?

Your physician will discuss the results of the test with you and your family after all of the data are received.

Will My Insurance Cover This Test?

Most health insurance companies will cover the test and the physician fee. The amount of coverage will vary from one company to another.

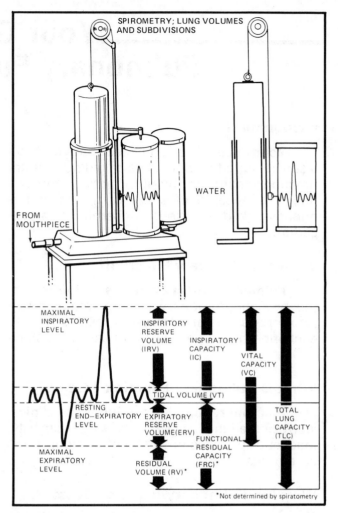

What pulmonary function tests measure.

Comments and Questions

Your Guide to
Chest Physiotherapy

Introduction

Your doctor has ordered a special treatment for you. It is called chest physiotherapy. In this information, many of the questions you may have concerning this treatment will be discussed.

What Is Chest Physiotherapy?

Chest physiotherapy is a mechanical method of percussing (patting) and vibrating the chest to effectively loosen and help drain secretions. **Postural drainage** (drainage of specific lung area by body positioning) is used along with percussion and vibration.

Why Is Chest Physiotherapy Done?

Chest physiotherapy is done to help move thick mucous secretions from areas deep in the lung to central airway passages. Then they can be removed more easily (by coughing, etc.).

Is There Any Preparation for This Procedure?

Yes!
1. Chest physiotherapy should not be done immediately after eating.

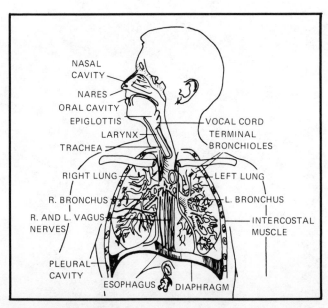

The respiratory system.

2. It will be scheduled early in the day or at a time when you may rest after the therapy.
3. You will want extra pillows and tissues at your bedside.
4. Chest physiotherapy may be done on an out-patient basis.

Where Is the Chest Physiotherapy Treatment Done?

These treatments are usually done at the patient's bedside. When treatment is done on an out-patient basis, physiotherapy may be done either in the respiratory department or in physical therapy department.

Who Will Do the Chest Physiotherapy Treatments?

These treatments will be done by highly trained technologists in respiratory or physical therapy departments, or by nurses who are trained in chest physiotherapy.

How Are the Treatments Given?

A nurse and therapist will come to your room. They will listen to your lung sounds. This will give an idea where most of the mucous problems are. They will then drape your chest with a towel and, standing opposite the site (area) requiring therapy, rhythmically clap the chest wall. Their hands will be in a cupped position. At regular intervals you will be asked to breathe deeply and cough. They will then continue to clap the chest wall, loosening the secretions. This is known as **chest percussion**. **Chest vibration** is done by placing one hand upon the other over the affected site. You will be asked to breathe in deeply and then exhale. The chest is vibrated by the technologist or nurse during expiration (breathing out). You will be given time to rest and cough between vibration cycles. Postural drainage is accomplished by physically positioning you to aid in respiratory drainage. You will be made as comfortable as possible in the position.

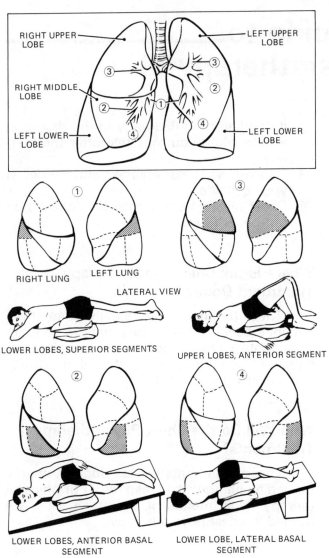

Positions for postural drainage.

When Will I Feel the Results From These Treatments?

You may feel results from the very first treatment by breathing more easily and by coughing up mucus that is causing the congestion.

Are There Any Side Effects From These Treatments?

Only good ones: Ability to cough up secretions more easily, being able to breathe more easily, and deeper.

Will My Insurance Cover These Treatments?

Most health insurance companies will cover the treatments. The amount of coverage will vary from one insurance company to another.

Your Guide to Chest X-Ray

Introduction

Your doctor has requested an X-ray of your chest. This information will discuss some of the questions you may have concerning the procedure.

What Is a Chest X-Ray?

A **chest X-ray** or **radiography** is a picture of the internal structures of the thoracic (chest) cavity.

Why Is a Chest X-Ray Done?

A chest X-ray is done to detect diseases of the chest; including pneumonia, other infectious processes, cancer, effusions (fluid), size and shape of organs, etc.

Is There Any Preparation for the Procedure?

No! This procedure is painless and it may be done on an out-patient as well as an in-patient basis. You will be asked to put on a hospital gown and to remove all jewelry.

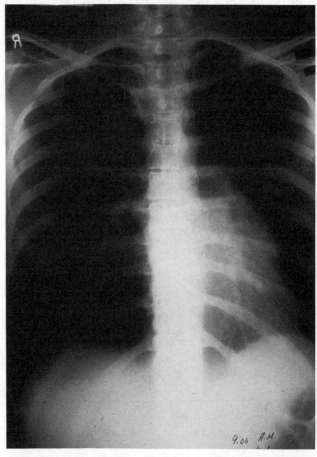

Actual chest X-ray. (By permission of the Radiology Dept., Lexington County Hospital, West Columbia, SC.)

Where Will the Procedure Be Done?

Chest X-rays may be done in a number of places, physician's office, clinics, X-ray department of a hospital, emergency room, patient's bedside, etc.

Who Will Do the Procedure?

The actual X-ray will be taken by a radiological technologist. The film will then be interpreted (read) by a radiologist. A **radiologist** is a physician who specializes in radiation and radioactive materials for the diagnosis and treatment of medical diseases.

How Is a Chest X-Ray Taken?

A chest X-ray is taken by positioning your chest against a photographic film, and expos-

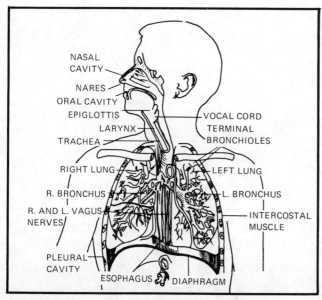

NASAL CAVITY
NARES
ORAL CAVITY
EPIGLOTTIS
LARYNX
TRACHEA
VOCAL CORD
TERMINAL BRONCHIOLES
RIGHT LUNG
LEFT LUNG
R. BRONCHUS
L. BRONCHUS
R. AND L. VAGUS NERVES
INTERCOSTAL MUSCLE
PLEURAL CAVITY
ESOPHAGUS
DIAPHRAGM

The respiratory system.

ing that film by the use of radiation. More than one view (position) may be needed for an accurate diagnosis.

When Will I Know the Results?

Your physician will inform you of the results after your film has been read by the radiologist.

Are There Any Complications or Side Effects?

No! As was stated previously, this procedure is painless, and quickly done. It is no more than an "inside" picture of your chest.

Will My Insurance Cover This Procedure?

Most insurance companies will cover a percentage of the X-ray as well as the physician fee. The amount of coverage will differ from company to company.

Comments and Questions

Your Guide to Bronchoscopy

Introduction

Your physician has requested that you have a special procedure done called a bronchoscopy. In this information, many of the questions you may have concerning the procedure will be discussed.

What Is Bronchoscopy?

A **bronchoscopy** is the inspection of the interior of the tracheobronchial tree (large air passage) by means of a **bronchoscope** (electrically lighted tube).

Why Is a Bronchoscopy Done?

A bronchoscopy is done for diagnostic purposes (collection of specimens for laboratory analysis) or therapeutic purposes (removal of foreign bodies from the respiratory tree).

Is There Any Preparation for This Procedure?

Yes.
1. Food is withheld until after the procedure.
2. You will be requested to put on a hospital gown.

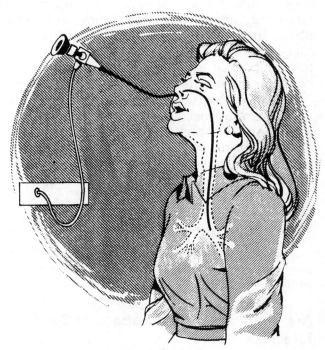

Diagram of bronchoscope insertion.

3. A small needle may be placed in your vein for fluid or medication.
4. You will be given medication to help you relax during the procedure. One of these medications may make your mouth dry.

Where Is the Procedure Done?

A bronchoscopy may be done in a respiratory unit or laboratory, X-ray department, or other specified areas of the hospital.

Who Will Do the Procedure?

This procedure, like many other procedures, utilizes the team approach. The team members will include a respiratory therapist, technologist, and a physician who specializes in diseases of the respiratory system.

How Is the Procedure Done?

You will be helped onto a table. The doctor will spray your throat with an anesthetic (numbing medicine). This is done for two reasons: 1) it numbs the throat region; and 2) it inhibits (prevents) the gag reflex. The **gag re-**

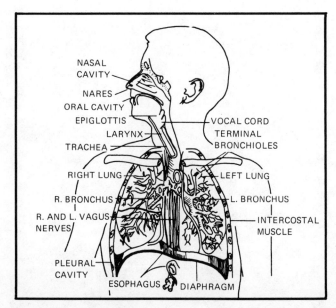

The respiratory system.

NASAL CAVITY
NARES
ORAL CAVITY
EPIGLOTTIS
LARYNX
TRACHEA
RIGHT LUNG
R. BRONCHUS
R. AND L. VAGUS NERVES
PLEURAL CAVITY
ESOPHAGUS
DIAPHRAGM
VOCAL CORD
TERMINAL BRONCHIOLES
LEFT LUNG
L. BRONCHUS
INTERCOSTAL MUSCLE

flex causes you to retch or to heave. The bronchoscope is then inserted. The physician may ask that the room lights be turned down. This allows the physician to see the light of the bronchoscope more clearly. Depending on the reason for the procedure, the physician may take a small piece of lung tissue or mucus for laboratory analysis, or may remove a foreign object (pennies, buttons, fluids, etc.) from the lung. There will be times that you may want to cough. It is important that you try not to cough or move. The bronchoscope is removed, and you will be returned to your room.

After the procedure, you will be very sleepy from the medication. You will not be given anything to eat or drink for 2 to 4 hours post procedure. This will ensure that the gag reflex has returned. A nurse will check you frequently. This is routine procedure.

When Will I Know the Results?

The physician will discuss the results with you and your family later that day or the next morning.

Are There Any Complications or Side Effects?

As in any procedure, there is always a slight chance of a complication occurring. However, the information gained from this procedure far outweighs not having the procedure done. Most common side effect is a sore throat post procedure.

Will My Insurance Cover the Procedure?

Most health insurance companies will cover the procedure and the physician fee. The amount of coverage will differ from one company to another.

Comments and Questions

Your Guide to Bronchography

Introduction

Your doctor has ordered a special test for you called bronchography. In this information, many of the questions you may have concerning this procedure will be discussed. You may hear this procedure referred to as a bronchogram.

What Is Bronchography?

Bronchography is an X-ray examination of the bronchial tree by the injection of a special dye.

What Is a Bronchogram?

A **bronchogram** is the X-ray obtained during bronchography.

Why Is Bronchography Done?

Bronchography is done to aid in the diagnosis of acute and chronic lung diseases.

Is There Any Preparation for the Procedure?

Yes!

1. You will not be allowed to have anything by mouth from midnight (day of the procedure) until after the procedure is over.

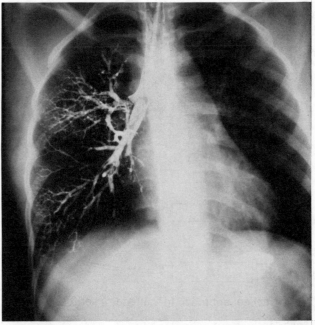

Bronchography showing dye in the lungs. (By permission of the Radiology Dept., Lexington County Hospital, West Columbia, SC.)

2. You will be asked to put on a hospital gown the day of the procedure.
3. A small needle will be inserted in a vein for use of intravenous fluids and/or medication.
4. Medication may be given prior to the procedure to help you relax.

Where Is Bronchography Done?

The bronchography procedure will be done in the radiology department.

Who Will Do the Bronchography Procedure?

The bronchography procedure will be done utilizing the team approach. The team members will consist of highly trained technologists and a radiologist. A **radiologist** is a physician who specializes in radiation and radioactive materials for medical diagnosis. The team may also include a physician who specializes in pulmonary problems.

How Is the Procedure Done?

You will be taken to the X-ray department and assisted onto a table. You will be made as

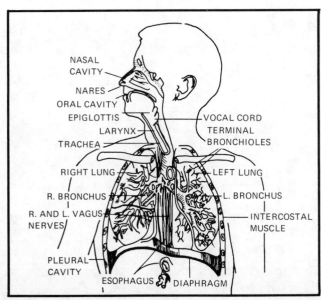

The respiratory system.

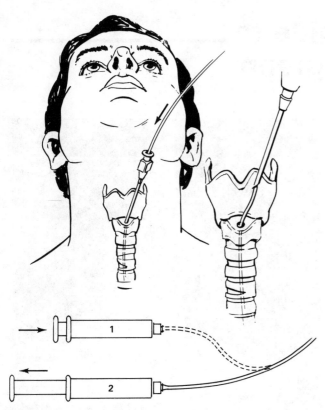

Trans-tracheal approach for catheter insertion.

When Will I Know the Results?

Your physician will talk to you and your family as soon as the X-ray report is received.

Are There Any Complications or Side Effects?

As in any procedure or test, there is always a slight chance of a complication occurring. However, the diagnostic benefits received from this procedure far outweigh the risk. Most common side effect is a sore throat post procedure.

Will My Insurance Cover This Procedure?

Most health insurance companies will cover the procedure as well as the physician fee. The amount of coverage will differ from one insurance company to another.

Comments and Questions

comfortable as possible. A pillow will be placed beneath your shoulders. This position will allow the head to fall back and the neck to become extended. From this point there are two methods, either of which may be used. The first method is to do a bronchoscopy and selectively **catheterize** (insert a small rubber tube) the area of the bronchial tree to be studied. Contrast media (dye) is then injected through the catheter. A **bronchoscopy** is the inspection of the interior of the tracheobronchial tree (air passages in the lung) by means of a bronchoscope (electrically lighted endoscope). The second method is to use the **transtracheal approach**. This is a procedure of catheterizing the tracheobronchial tree by means of a catheter inserted via a needle through the cricothyroid membrane located in the neck. The contrast media will again be injected through the catheter.

Whichever method is used, you will have a feeling of wanting to cough when the dye is injected. This is a normal reflex. Try not to cough while the X-rays are being taken. At the end of the procedure, the catheter and the majority of the contrast media are removed.

After the procedure, you will be returned to your room to rest. A nurse will check you frequently. This is normal routine.

Your Guide to
Thoracentesis
(Pleural Fluid Analysis)

Introduction

Your doctor has requested you have a special test performed called thoracentesis. In this information, many of the questions you may have concerning this procedure will be discussed.

What Is Thoracentesis?

Thoracentesis is a procedure performed to remove fluid or air from the pleural space (space between chest wall and lung).

Why Is Thoracentesis Done?

Thoracentesis may be done for diagnostic or therapeutic reasons. Diagnostically, a thoracentesis is done to obtain fluid for laboratory analysis. Therapeutically, a thoracentesis is done to relieve **dyspnea** (difficulty in breathing), **hypoxemia** (decrease in O_2 in blood) by fluid withdrawal, or to instill medication into the pleural space.

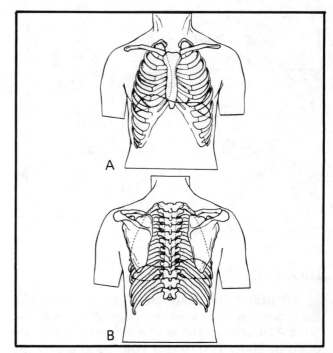

Outlines of the pleural spaces.

Is There Any Preparation For Thoracentesis?

Yes!
1. You will be requested to put on a hospital gown.
2. Food will be withheld until after the procedure.
3. If you do not already have an IV, a small needle will be inserted into your vein for fluids, and/or medication.
4. Medication may be given prior to the procedure to help you relax.

Where Is the Procedure Performed?

Thoracentesis is usually done in an examination room, special procedure area, or it may be done at the patient's bedside.

Who Will Do the Procedure?

The thoracentesis procedure will be done by a physician and nurse who have had training in the procedure.

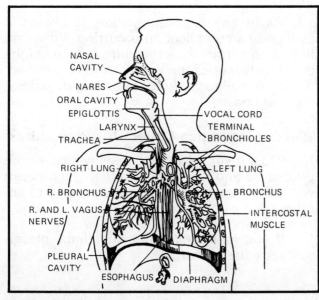

NASAL CAVITY
NARES
ORAL CAVITY
EPIGLOTTIS
LARYNX
TRACHEA
RIGHT LUNG
R. BRONCHUS
R. AND L. VAGUS NERVES
PLEURAL CAVITY
ESOPHAGUS
DIAPHRAGM
VOCAL CORD
TERMINAL BRONCHIOLES
LEFT LUNG
L. BRONCHUS
INTERCOSTAL MUSCLE

The respiratory system.

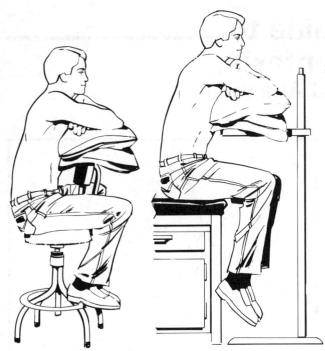

Positions for thoracentesis.

How Is the Procedure Done?

You may be asked to sit on the edge of a table or bed with your legs dangling over the side. A bedside stand with a pillow on it is often used to allow you to rest your head and arms on it while in a sitting position. The sitting position is necessary to ensure that the diaphragm (lower chest muscle) is as low as possible.

A second position that may be used is sitting in a straight back chair, facing the back of the chair. The back of the chair, draped with a pillow, can then be used to support your head and arms.

The area to be entered is then washed with an antiseptic (germ-killing) solution and a sterile (germ-free) field established, using sterile towels and sheets. It is *very* important that

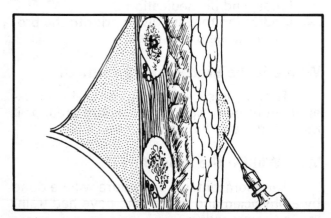

Insertion of anesthetic solution.

you *do not touch* these sterile towels and sheets. They have been placed over the area to aid in the prevention of an infection. The physician, with the help of X-ray and/or ultrasound, has been able to localize the area in which the needle is to be placed.

The next step is to **infiltrate**, or inject the area, with a numbing medication (anesthetic) like the dentist uses. This may burn, but it will last only a few seconds. The aspirating needle (or trocar system as it is often called) is then inserted until pleural fluid is obtained. (The physician may ask you to hold your breath while he is inserting the needle.) The fluid is withdrawn slowly and a specimen is sent to the laboratory for analysis. If a great deal of fluid is noted, a chest tube may be inserted for continuous drainage. If only a small amount of fluid is obtained, the needle is withdrawn (again you may be asked to hold your breath), and the area cleaned with an antiseptic solution. The site is then covered with a sterile dressing. A pressure dressing may be used to prevent any air leakage.

After the procedure, you will be checked frequently by a nurse. This is normal practice. Your vital signs (blood pressure, pulse, and respiration), as well as the procedure site will be checked.

When Will I Know the Results?

After the procedure is over, and the laboratory results have been received, the physician will talk to you and your family.

Are There Any Complications or Side Effects?

As in any procedure, there is always a chance of a complication occurring. However, the benefit from the procedure far outweighs the risk. A few of the complications that may occur are collapsed lung, infection, or pulmonary edema.

Will My Insurance Cover This Procedure?

Most insurance companies will cover the procedure and the physician fee. The amount will differ from one insurance company to another.

If you have any other questions, please contact your doctor.

Your Guide to
Needle Biopsy of the Lung

Introduction

Your doctor has ordered a special test for you called a needle biopsy of the lung. In this information, many of the questions you may have concerning this test will be discussed.

What Is a Needle Biopsy of the Lung?

A **needle biopsy** of the lung is the procedure of obtaining a small piece of lung tissue by means of a needle passed through the chest wall. This is known as the **transthoracic** (across the chest wall) approach.

Why Is a Needle Biopsy Done?

A needle biopsy may be done to aid in the diagnosis of pleural effusions, pleural disease, pneumonia, cancer, fungal disease, etc. The diagnosis is determined by obtaining a small piece of lung tissue for histologic (study of tissue), cytologic (study of cells), or bacteriologic (study of bacteria and fungus) analysis.

Is There Any Preparation For the Procedure?

Yes.
1. Food will be withheld until after the procedure.

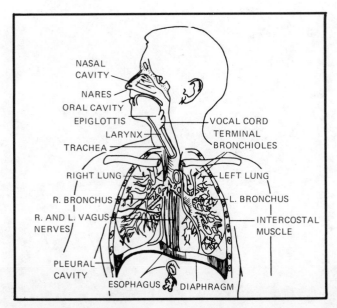

The respiratory system.

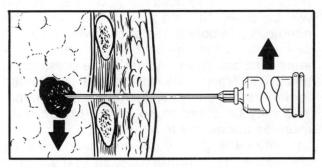

Needle inserted into lung tissue.

2. You will be requested to put on a hospital gown.
3. You may be given some medication to help you to relax for the test.
4. This test may be done on an outpatient basis. You will be asked to stay 2 to 4 hours after the procedure is completed to be checked for any side effects, and to rest.

Where Is the Procedure Done?

This procedure may be done in several areas of the hospital (treatment rooms, respiratory department, X-ray department, special procedure areas, patient's bedside, etc.). This procedure is made easier when a fluoroscopy unit (X-ray) is used.

Who Will Do the Procedure?

This procedure will utilize a team approach. The team members will include nurses, technologists, and a physician. All of the team members have been trained in this procedure.

How Is the Procedure Done?

You will be taken to a procedure room with an X-ray machine called a fluoroscope. A member of the medical team will help you onto the table. The physician will tell you whether to lie down in the prone (face down) or supine (face up) position. The physician will mark the area to be entered with a pen. This area was determined by previous X-rays and initial fluoroscopy. This area is now washed with an antiseptic (germ-killing) solution. A sterile (germ-free) field is established with the use of sterile towels and sheets. It is *very important* that you *do not touch* these towels or sheets. At this point the physician will anesthetize (numb) the skin around the area where the needle will be inserted. This may burn, but it will last only a few seconds. With the aid of fluoroscopy, the physician will insert the needle into the affected area. While positioning the needle, you will be asked to hold your breath. Once the needle is positioned, the doctor will connect a syringe to it, and pull back on the syringe, creating suction. You may feel some pressure at this point. When sufficient material is obtained for laboratory analysis, the needle is removed. You may be asked to hold your breath once more as the needle is removed.

After the procedure, your lungs will be checked with the fluoroscope, and a dry, sterile dressing placed over the site. You will be returned to your room where you may sleep for a while from the medication you were given. A nurse will check you frequently for a few hours. This is a routine procedure.

When Will I Know the Results?

It may take 12 to 24 hours to obtain the laboratory data. The physician will talk to you and your family after receiving all of the data.

Are There Any Complications or Side Effects?

As in any procedure there is always a slight chance of a complication occurring. However, the information obtained from the procedure far outweighs not having the procedure done. Two complications which may occur are infection or a **pneumothorax** (collapsed lung).

Will My Insurance Cover This Procedure?

Most health insurance companies will cover the procedure as well as the physician fee. The amount of coverage will differ from one company to another.

Comments and Questions

Your Guide to
Closed Thoracostomy

Introduction

Your doctor has ordered the insertion of a chest tube. Many times the need for insertion of a chest tube is an emergency situation. This information will discuss many of the questions you may have concerning the procedure.

What Is a Closed Thoracostomy by Means of a Chest Tube?

This is a procedure that drains the pleural space by means of a tube placed between the ribs and through the chest wall (transthoracic approach) into the pleural space.

Where Is the Pleural Space?

The **pleural space** is formed between two layers of pleura membranes. One layer lines the chest wall and one layer is the outer covering of the lungs. In this space there is a very tiny amount of fluid (4 cc) to lubricate the two membranes. More important is the fact that there is always a fluctuating *negative* intrapleural pressure.

Why Is a Chest Tube Inserted?

There are several indications (reasons) for the insertion of a chest tube. The following are

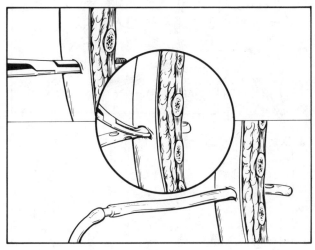

Thoracostomy tube inserted into chest wall.

a few of the indications: **hemothorax** (blood in the lung); **pneumothorax** (collapsed lung due to fluid or air); **empyema** (pus in the lung); **pleural effusion** (build-up of fluid in the pleural spaces), and chest trauma.

Is There Any Preparation for a Chest Tube?

Yes!
1. Food will be withheld until after the procedure.
2. You will be asked to put on a hospital gown.
3. If you do not have an IV, a nurse will put a small needle into your vein to be used for fluids or medication.
4. You may be given some medication to help you relax.

Where Will the Procedure Be Done?

The insertion of a chest tube may be done almost anywhere in the hospital setting. The most frequently used areas are emergency room, operating room, critical care units, X-ray department, and respiratory units.

Who Will Do the Procedure?

The insertion of a chest tube is usually done by a surgeon or surgical resident and a nurse who have had training in this procedure.

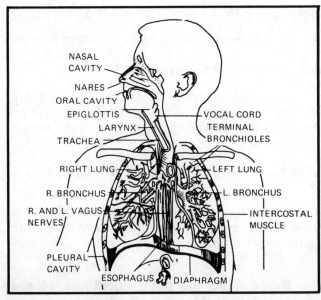

The respiratory system.

NASAL CAVITY
NARES
ORAL CAVITY
EPIGLOTTIS
LARYNX
TRACHEA
RIGHT LUNG
R. BRONCHUS
R. AND L. VAGUS NERVES
PLEURAL CAVITY
ESOPHAGUS
DIAPHRAGM
VOCAL CORD
TERMINAL BRONCHIOLES
LEFT LUNG
L. BRONCHUS
INTERCOSTAL MUSCLE

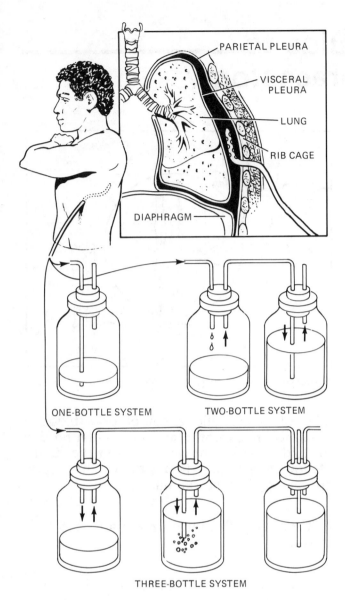

PARIETAL PLEURA

VISCERAL PLEURA

LUNG

RIB CAGE

DIAPHRAGM

ONE-BOTTLE SYSTEM   TWO-BOTTLE SYSTEM

THREE-BOTTLE SYSTEM

Connection of tube to drainage system.

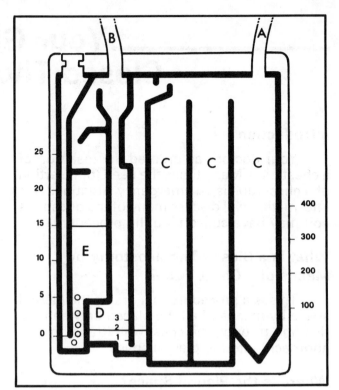

Disposable drainage system.

How Is the Procedure Done?

You will be requested to lie on your back on a table or in bed. The physician, by looking at your chest X-rays, will decide in which area to insert the chest tube. If air is the cause of the problem the tube will be inserted in the 2nd intercostal space. If fluid is the problem, it will be the 8th intercostal space. A nurse will clean the area with an antiseptic (germ-killing) solution and establish a sterile (germ-free) field with sterile towels and sheets. It is very important that you *do not touch* these sterile towels and sheets. The physician will now inject the area with a numbing medication (anesthetic). This may sting, but it will last only a few seconds. Now the physician will insert a tube between the ribs into the chest cavity. You may feel pressure at this time, and you may

be asked to hold your breath. The tube is clamped so that no air can enter the chest cavity. The tube is secured in place by sutures and tape. The area is cleaned and covered with a dry sterile dressing. The chest tube will now be connected to a special suction system that will draw the air or fluid from your chest. This does not hurt.

After the procedure, nurses will check you very often. They will pinch the chest tube to help keep the fluid or air moving out of your chest. This is called milking the tube.

How Long Will I Need to Have the Tube?

The average length of time is 3 to 5 days.

Are There Any Complications?

As in any procedure there is always a slight chance of a complication occurring. However, the benefit to you of having the procedure done far outweighs the risk.

Will My Insurance Cover This Procedure?

Most health insurance companies will cover the procedure and the physician fee. The amount of coverage will differ from one company to another.

If you have any other questions, please contact your doctor.

rointestinal Studies

wel Series

en an esophagography per GI series. A barium consists of a cineradin) examination of the ic examination of the s usually done as a part dicated in patients who regurgitating. The upes is an examination of nd small intestine after um by the patient. This who present with dysic burning or bleeding, es.
are done to aid in the strictures, varices, moulcers, malabsorption GI problems.

Nurse's Responsibilities

Pre-Test
1. Explain procedure to patient and family.
2. Tell patient to be on a low-residue diet for 48 to 72 hours prior to the test. Explain what a low-residue diet consists of and why it is important.
3. Patient will be NPO the night of the study until after it is complete.
4. Patient should be asked *not* to smoke the night or morning of the test.
5. Inform the patient that the procedure is done in stages and may take 4 to 6 hours to complete.
6. A warm saline or tap water enema along with a cathartic is ordered the evening prior to the study.
7. Have the patient put on a hospital gown and remove all jewelry that is in the way.
8. Have patient void prior to starting the procedure.
9. Explain to the patient that he or she will be placed into many positions during the study, and it is important not to move during the time the X-rays are being made.
10. Explain that the barium is thick and chalky, that it may not taste good, but he or she will have to drink about 300 to 600 ml of it.
11. This may be done on an out-patient basis.
12. No alcoholic beverages should be consumed 24 hours prior to the test.

Precautions
1. Medications that are anticholinergic and/or narcotics are withheld for 24 hours due to their effect on small bowel motility.
2. This procedure is contraindicated in patients with symptoms of perforation or obstruction of the gastrointestinal tract.

Post-Procedure
1. Make patient comfortable and encourage bed rest.
2. If all radiographs have been taken, the patient may eat, drink, and resume medications.
3. Check orders. It is common to give the patient a laxative or enema post study to aid in the evacuation of the barium.

Lower GI Study (Barium Enema)

A barium enema is a radiographic examination of the large intestine, after barium sulfate (contrast media) has been instilled in the patient via a rectal tube. Often times, an air contrast study (double contrast) may be done simultaneously with the barium study (single contrast). These studies are indicated in patients presenting with symptoms of blood, pus, or mucous in the stool, lower abdominal pain, or altered bowel habits. Patients with ileostomies or colostomies may have the test to follow pathological process.

The main purpose of this examination is to aid in the diagnosis of diverticula inflammatory processes, cancer, polyps, and miscellaneous structural changes in the large intestine.

It is important that this procedure is done prior to the upper GI or barium swallow since it may take quite some time to rid the GI tract of the barium.

Nurse's Responsibilities

Pre-Test
1. Explain the procedure to the patient and family (may be done as an out-patient).
2. Follow the prescribed diet and bowel prep used by your hospital. This normally consists of (1) a low-residue diet from 24 to 72 hours prior to the examination; (2) castor oil the afternoon prior to the test; (3) clear liquids for the evening meal prior to the test; (4) cleansing enema the evening prior to the test or the morning of the test

(repeat enemas until clear); and (5) a light breakfast 1 hour prior to the test.
3. Encourage the patient to drink water 12 to 24 hours prior to the test. This aids in adequate hydration of the patient.
4. Have patient put on a hospital gown.
5. Ask patient to void prior to the test.
6. Warn patient of some cramping when the barium and air are inserted. Deep, slow breaths will help relieve cramping.
7. Instruct the patient to retain the enema until he or she is told to expel it.
8. Reassure the patient that he or she will be covered during the procedure and that he or she will be helped to turn.

Precautions
1. This test is contraindicated in patients with symptoms of cardiac dysrhythmia (tachycardia), obstruction or perforation of lower GI tract, and ulcerative colitis with megacolon or systemic toxicity.
2. Great care should be taken with patients demonstrating inflammatory processes, vascular insufficiency of the large intestine, and other *acute* large intestinal disease processes.
3. Improper bowel preparation will negate the study.
4. It is important that the barium enema is done prior to barium swallow or upper GI studies due to interference of contrast media.

Post-Procedure
1. Make patient comfortable, encourage rest.
2. After all radiographs have been taken, the patient may eat, drink, and resume medications.
3. Encourage fluid intake to assure proper hydration.
4. Check chart for orders on post procedure laxative and/or enema.

Insertion of a Nasogastric Tube

The insertion of a nasogastric tube is a fairly common procedure in most hospitals. Diagnostically, the tube may be inserted to aspirate gastric contents for laboratory analysis, and to decompress the stomach. Therapeutically, the nasogastric tube may be inserted to remove toxic contents (drugs, chemicals, etc.), to ice lavage to control bleeding, and for tube feedings, gastric or intestinal.

Nurse's Responsibilities

Pre-Test
1. Explain the procedure to the patient and family.
2. Inform the patient that the passage of the tube is uncomfortable but not painful.
3. Instruct the patient to sit up straight in a high Fowler's position.
4. Provide the patient with tissues, an emesis basin, ice chips, or a glass of water with a straw.

5. Instruct the patient that when he or she feels the tube in the back of the throat, to pant and to swallow. The ice chips or sips of water help the swallowing mechanism. If on NPO, have patient dry swallow.
7. Inform the patient that the tube will be secured to his or her face with tape, and that the nose will be lubricated so the tube will not rub.

Precautions
1. If the tube does not advance easily, stop and try the other side.
2. If the patient is uncooperative or has a very active gag reflex, ask the physician for a sedative order before trying to insert the tube again.
3. If specimens are obtained, label correctly and send to laboratory.

Post-Procedure
1. Make the patient as comfortable as possible.
2. Check the chart for orders. They will vary greatly depending upon why the tube was inserted.
3. Allow the patient time to relax.
4. If permitted, ask the patient's family to bring in hard candy. Hard candy will keep the patient's throat from getting sore.

Insertion of an Intestinal Tube

The insertion of an intestinal tube, like that of a nasogastric tube, may be done for diagnostic or therapeutic reasons. Diagnostically, the intestinal tube may be inserted to obtain an intestinal contents specimen for analysis. Therapeutically, it is used for relief of bowel obstruction and for intestinal tube feeding.

Types of Intestinal Tubes
Kaslow—Bowel obstruction and intestinal aspiration.

Cantor—Bowel obstruction and intestinal aspiration.

Dobbhoff—Intestinal feeding.

Hodge—Intestinal, pancreatic, biliary secretion.

Keofeed Silicone—Gastric or intestinal feeding.

Miller Abbot—Bowel obstruction and intestinal aspiration.

Keofeed Mercury—Gastric or intestinal feeding.

Nurse's Responsibilities

Pre-Test
1. Explain the procedure to the patient and family.
2. Inform the patient that passing the tube may be uncomfortable but is not painful.
3. Have the patient put on a hospital gown.
4. Explain to the patient that usually some medication is given to help the patient relax prior to the start of the procedure.

5. Food and liquids are withheld several hours prior to the insertion of the intestinal tube.
6. Position patient upright in bed in high Fowler's position.
7. Provide the patient with tissues, emesis basin and ice chips or a glass of water with a straw.
8. Explain to the patient when he or she feels the tube in the back of the throat, to pant and take a sip of water to facilitate the movement of the tube to the stomach.
9. Bend patient's chin to the chest. This also facilitates the passage of the tube to the stomach.
10. When the tube is in the stomach, position the patient on the right side. This will facilitate the passage of the tube to the small intestine.
11. Every hour, the tube is advanced 2–3" until the correct position is obtained. The position is documented by aspiration and X-ray.

Precautions
1. Have suction ready in case the patient begins to vomit.
2. Great care should be taken in this procedure in patients who are suspected to be perforated or who have an acute disease process.
3. Label all specimens and send to laboratory for analysis.

Post-Procedure
1. Make patient as comfortable as possible.
2. Allow the patient time to relax and rest.
3. Lubricate the nostril through which the tube passes.
4. Tape tube safely and securely to face.
5. Give analgesics as per order.
6. Hard candy, if allowed, may be used to moisten the throat.

Gastroscopy

A more appropriate term for this procedure is *esophagogastroduodenoscopy*. The definition of this procedure would then be the direct visualization of the mucosa of the esophagus, stomach, and duodenum utilizing a flexible fiberoptic endoscope.

This procedure is indicated in patients with upper GI bleeding, upper gastric pain, and in post-surgical patients with continued or recurrent symptoms.

This procedure is done diagnostically to evaluate structure or tissue abnormalities, to aid in the diagnosis of tumors (benign and maligant), ulcers, and inflammatory disease, and to obtain gastric specimens for laboratory analysis. Therapeutically, this procedure is done to remove foreign bodies from the upper GI system.

Nurse's Responsibilities

Pre-Test
1. Explain the procedure to the patient and family (may be done as an out-patient).

2. Check to see if a permit has been signed. If not, have one signed and witnessed.
3. Inform the patient that he or she will be NPO 6 to 12 hours prior to the test.
4. Ask the patient to put on a hospital gown.
5. If the patient has dentures, they should be removed prior to the procedure.
6. Check the chart and ask if the patient is allergic to any medications or local anesthetics.
7. Inform patient that he or she will have some medication to help relax prior to the procedure.
8. Check IV for signs of infiltration. If patient does not have an IV, start one with an 18g or greater size needle.
9. Explain to the patient that the throat will be sprayed with an anesthetic so that he or she will not feel the tube pass.
10. Inform patient that a feeling of pressure in the stomach is normal during the procedure.
11. Have patient void prior to the procedure.
12. Assist in getting the patient and chart ready for transfer to the procedure area.
13. Pre-medicate patient as per order on call for the procedure.

Precautions
1. This procedure is contraindicated in patients with known or suspected aortic aneurysm or perforated ulcer.
2. This procedure should be done prior to an upper GI series. Barium would interfere with visability of the mucosa.
3. If biopsies or specimens are obtained, label them properly and send them to the laboratory for analysis.
4. Emergency equipment and medications should be accessible to the procedure area.

Post-Procedure
1. Monitor vital signs q15 min × 4, q30 min × 4, q1 hr × 4, and q4 hr.
2. Observe patient for signs and symptoms of gastric perforation.
3. Withhold food and liquids until the gag reflex has returned.
4. Explain to the patient that a sore throat is normal for 24 to 72 hours post procedure.
5. Check the IV site for signs of infiltration.
6. Administer analgesics as per order for discomfort.

Proctosigmoidoscopy

Proctosigmoidoscopy is the internal inspection of the anal canal, rectum, and the distal sigmoid colon. This procedure comprises three parts: (1) a digital examination; (2) sigmoidoscopy utilizing a sigmoidoscope; and (3) proctoscopy utilizing a proctoscope.

This procedure is indicated in patients who have rectal bleeding, lower GI pain, change in bowel habits, or pus and/or mucus in the stool.

Diagnostically, this procedure is done (1) to aid in the diagnosis of tumors (malignant and benign), hemorrhoids, polyps, fissures, fistulas, abscesses within the anal canal or rectum, and (2) to aid in the diagnosis of ulcerative or inflammatory bowel disease.

Nurse's Responsibilities

Pre-Test
1. Explain the procedure to the patient and family (may be done as an out-patient).
2. Explain the knee-chest or the lateral position. Inform the patient that two tubes will be passed. The procedure is not painful but can be uncomfortable.
3. Inform the patient that if he or she will cooperate with the doctor, the test will proceed smoothly.
4. Explain that the patient may experience the urge to defecate upon insertion of the tubes, and may feel cramping and muscle spasm at times throughout the study. All of these feelings are normal and taking deep breaths will help to relax the muscles.
5. Check the chart to see that a permit has been signed. If not, have one signed and witnessed.
6. Have patient follow the orders for bowel preparation for this procedure. These procedures differ from one hospital and physician to another.
7. Clear liquids are usually ordered 24 to 48 hours prior to the procedure.
8. Have patient put on a hospital gown.
9. A tap water enema may be given 2 to 3 hours prior to the test.
10. Have patient void prior to the procedure.
11. Prepare the patient and chart for transport to the procedure area.
12. In rare instances, pre-medication may be given.

Precautions
1. If barium study has been done recently, this will interfere with visibility of mucosa.
2. Poor bowel preparation will interfere with procedure.
3. If biopsies or other specimens have been obtained, correctly label and send to laboratory for analysis.

Post-Procedure
1. Make patient comfortable.
2. If patient is passing flatus, give him or her some privacy.
3. Order a meal tray or snack if patient missed a meal.
4. Explain that, if patient had a biopsy taken, a small amount of blood in the stool is normal.
5. Observe patient for signs and symptoms of bowel perforation, bleeding, abdominal distension or pain. If these symptoms do present themselves, notify the physician.

Oral Cholecystography

Oral cholecystography is a radiographic examination of the gallbladder after the ingestion of an iodinated contrast dye.

It is indicated in patients who have symptoms of gallbladder disease (right upper quadrant pain, intolerance to fat, nausea, and jaundice).

The purpose of this radiographic procedure is to aid in the diagnosis of gallstones, inflammatory process and tumors.

Nurse's Responsibilities

Pre-Test
1. Explain the procedure to the patient and family.
2. If ordered, give the patient a high-fat content meal at noon the day prior to the test.
3. The evening meal will be very low-fat content.
4. Patient will be NPO from evening meal to after the procedure except for water.
5. Give the patient the ordered number of contrast pills 2 to 3 hours past dinner. Ensure the patient is *not* sensitive to iodine. Patient should now be NPO except for water.
6. Have the patient put on a hospital gown.
7. The morning of the test, give the patient a cleansing enema if ordered.
8. Notify physician and X-ray if patient vomited any of the dye tablets.

Precautions
1. This procedure should not be done until several days post barium study, because of interference of visability.
2. Contraindicated in iodine hypersensitivity.
3. Extreme caution in performing this procedure in patients with renal or liver disease.
4. Procedure area should have emergency equipment and medications immediately available.
5. Failure to adhere to dietary procedure can lead to false results.
6. Poor bowel preparation can hinder visibility.

Post-Procedure
1. Check chart:
   a. If tests are negative, the patient may eat and resume previous orders.
   b. If tests results are positive, the physician may want to keep the patient on a low-fat diet or NPO.
2. Allow patient time to rest from procedure.

Intravenous and T-Tube Cholangiography

Intravenous and T-tube cholangiography are radiographic and tomographic examinations of the biliary tree. Utilizing the intravenous route for the contrast media in the intravenous cholangiography and the T-tube in the T-tube cholangiography, the biliary tree is opacified in patients who have had cholecystectomies.

In very rare circumstances, the intravenous route may be utilized for examination of the gallbladder. This procedure is indicated in those patients who cannot absorb the normal oral contrast agents.

The purpose of these procedures is to aid in the diagnosis of calculi, strictures, congenital abnormalities, fistulas, and neoplasms in the biliary tree.

Nurse's Responsibilities

Pre-Test
1. Explain procedures to patient and family (may be done as an out-patient).
2. Check to make sure a permit has been signed. If not, have one signed and witnessed.
3. Inform IV cholangiography patient that he or she must maintain a low-residue diet 24 to 48 hours prior to the study, and a meal high in simple fats the evening prior to the study.
4. Check the chart and ask if patient is allergic to iodine, shellfish, or has had a prior reaction to contrast media.
5. Check the patient's IV for patency and signs of infiltration. If the patient does not have an IV, start one with an 18g or greater needle.
6. Follow the bowel preparation ordered by the physician. Often this will include a cleansing enema the morning of the procedure.
7. For the patient who will be having the T-tube cholangiography procedure, the physician may order the T-tube clamped for 24 hours prior to the procedure.
8. Inform the patient that he or she may experience nausea, vomiting, perspiring, urticaria, or rarely, anaphylaxis, upon insertion of the dye. The T-tube patient also may feel some pressure in the right upper quadrant.
9. Patients are normally NPO prior to the study to aid in bile concentration.
10. Assist the patient into a hospital gown.
11. Ask patient to void prior to procedure.
12. Ensure that the patient and chart are ready for transport to the X-ray department.

Precautions
1. Hepatic and renal disease (acute or chronic) are contraindications for this procedure.
2. Hypersensitivity to iodine is a contraindication in this study. However, if the study *must* be done, the patient should first be prepped with steroids.
3. Test results may be false or invalidated due to poor bowel preparation, dietary preparation, or air (T-tube patient) over the bile ducts obstructing the view.
4. Procedure area should have emergency medications and equipment available.

Post-Procedure
1. Make patient comfortable and allow time to rest post procedure.

2. Check chart for pertinent orders and to ensure *all* radiographs are complete.
3. Order meal tray or snack for patient if procedure is complete.
4. Observe patient for signs of delayed contrast reaction.
5. If T-tube has been removed, check site for drainage.
6. If T-tube has not been removed, check chart for orders regarding opening it up to straight drainage or clamping.

Abdominal Paracentesis

An abdominal paracentesis is a percutaneous puncture of the abdominal cavity. Diagnostically, this procedure is done to obtain peritoneal fluid for laboratory analysis and to assess abdominal injury due to trauma. Therapeutically, this procedure may be done to relieve urinary urgency or dyspnea due to fluid accumulation.

Nurse's Responsibilities

Pre-Test
1. Explain the procedure to the patient and family.
2. Check the chart to see that a permit has been signed. If not, get one signed and witnessed.
3. Check the patient's IV for patency and signs of infiltration. If patient does not have an IV, start one with an 18g or larger needle.
4. Have the patient put on a hospital gown.
5. Have patient void before procedure.
6. Place the patient in a high Fowler's position, feet flat on the floor, and the peritoneum exposed.
7. Explain to the patient that the physician will numb the puncture site. It may sting but should not be painful.
8. Give emotional support to the patient.
9. Assist physician with tap.
10. Label specimens correctly and send to laboratory for analysis.

Precautions
1. Extreme care should be given to patients who have a known bleeding problem, or who are critically ill.
2. Observe patient for signs and symptoms of shock due to rapid withdrawal of fluid.
3. If the patient is on antibiotics, note this on the laboratory slips.

Post-Procedure Care
1. Make patient comfortable.
2. Monitor vital signs q15 min × 4, q30 min × 4, q1 hr × 4, and q4 hr.
3. Observe puncture site dressing for drainage. Reinforce if necessary.
4. Observe for signs and symptoms of shock and/or hemorrhage. Notify physician immediately.

5. Check patient for abdominal distension and pain that may denote perforation of small or large intestine. Notify physician immediately.
6. Check IV for patency and signs of infiltration.
7. Monitor urinary output, observe for hematuria.
8. Check chart for pertinent fluid and medication orders.

Percutaneous Liver Biopsy

A percutaneous liver biopsy is the excision of a piece of liver tissue by a hollow needle through the abdominal wall.

A liver biopsy is indicated in those patients with known or suspected liver tumor (benign or malignant) or cirrhosis of the liver.

The purpose of the procedure is to obtain a minute amount of liver tissue for laboratory analysis to aid in the diagnosis of liver infections, neoplasm, and parenchymal disease.

Nurse's Responsibilities

Pre-Test
1. Explain the procedure to the patient and family.
2. Check chart for a signed permit. If one has not been signed, obtain the written permit and witness it.
3. Check the chart to see if a recent coagulation study has been done.
4. Patient is usually NPO 6 to 8 hours prior to the study.
5. Check the IV for patency and signs of infiltration. If the patient does not have an IV, start one with an 18g or larger needle.
6. Have patient put on a hospital gown.

7. Ask patient to void prior to the procedure.
8. Give pre-medication as per order on call for the procedure.
9. Position patient on left side with a pillow under the head and right shoulder.
10. Assist physician in establishing a sterile field.
11. Inform the patient that the numbing medicine will sting but there should be no pain.
12. Explain to the patient the importance of not moving and holding his or her breath when asked.
13. Label all specimens correctly and send them to laboratory for analysis.
14. Apply pressure dressing to puncture site.

Precautions
1. This procedure is contraindicated in patients with a bleeding problem.
2. Patient may experience right shoulder pain due to the close proximity of the phrenic nerve.
3. It is necessary to have patient hold his or her breath to stop movement of chest wall.

Post-Procedure
1. Position patient on his or her right side and make as comfortable as possible. (Some physicians place a small sand bag under right costal margin to ensure hemostasis.)
2. Patient may resume prior diet.
3. Bed rest for 12 to 24 hours post procedure is usual.
4. Monitor vital signs q15 min ×4, q30 min ×4, q1 hr ×4, q4 hr.
5. Observe for signs and symptoms of hemorrhage, pneumothorax, or peritonitis. Notify physician immediately.
6. Administer analgesics as per order for puncture site discomfort.

Your Guide to
Upper GI & Small Bowel Series

Introduction

Your doctor has ordered a special X-ray procedure (test) for you. It is called an upper GI (gastrointestinal) study. In this information, you will find a discussion of many of the questions you may have concerning this procedure.

What Is an Upper GI Study?

An **upper GI study** is an X-ray of the esophagus (tube connecting the mouth to the stomach), the stomach, and the first section of the small intestine called the duodenum.

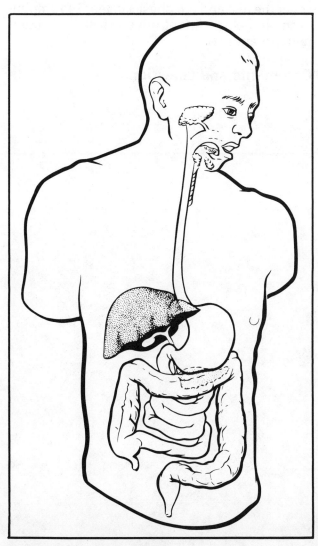

The gastrointestinal system.

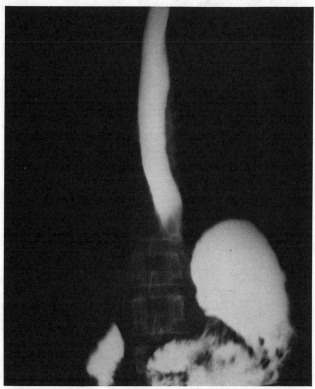

Normal esophagus shown with barium dye. (By permission of the Radiology Dept., Lexington County Hospital, West Columbia, SC.)

Why Is an Upper GI Study Done?

An upper GI study aids in the medical diagnosis of tumors, varices (large, damaged veins), and lesions of the upper GI tract.

Is an Upper GI Study and Barium Swallow the Same Test?

No! A barium swallow is the recording on X-ray film of actually swallowing the barium (dye). This test is done when the physician is looking for problems that involve the esophagus.

Is There Any Preparation for the Upper GI Study?

Yes!
1. Do not drink any alcoholic beverages (including wine or beer) the day before the procedure.
2. After midnight of the day of the test, *do not* eat or drink anything until the test is over.

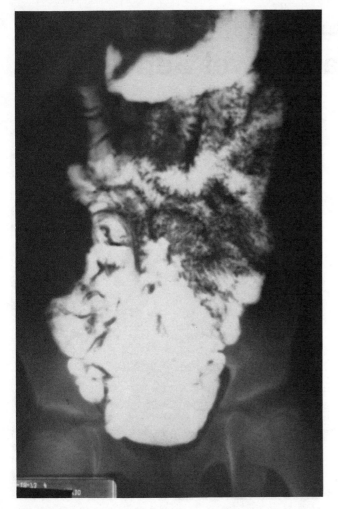

Stomach and small bowel. (By permission of the Radiology Dept., Lexington County Hospital, West Columbia, SC.)

3. You will be asked to put on a hospital gown.
4. This procedure may be done on an out-patient basis.

Where Is the Upper GI Study Done?

The upper GI study is done in a special room (fluoroscopic-type of X-ray) in the radiology (X-ray) department.

Who Will Do the Upper GI Study?

The upper GI study utilizes the team approach. The team consists of highly trained technologists and a radiologist. A **radiologist** is a physician who specializes in the use of radiation and radioactive materials for medical diagnosis.

How Is the Upper GI Study Done?

You will be taken to the X-ray department, where you will be asked to swallow a glass of barium. Barium is a flavored (strawberry or chocolate malt), chalky fluid that is radiopaque (can be seen by X-ray). X-ray pictures will then be taken while you are standing in front of and lying on the X-ray table. It is very important that you stay still while each X-ray picture is taken.

After the procedure, you will return to your room, or if you are an out-patient, you may return home. You will now be able to eat and drink. Your doctor will order a mild laxative for you. This laxative will help you get rid of the barium from your GI tract.

When Will I Know the Results of the Study?

When your doctor receives the report of your test, you and your family will be told the results of the study.

Will My Insurance Cover This Test?

Most health insurance companies will cover the test and the physician fee. The amount of coverage will differ from one insurance company to another.

Comments and Questions

Your Guide to Lower GI Study (Barium Enema)

Introduction

Your doctor has ordered a special X-ray test for you called a lower GI study or barium enema. In this information, many of the questions you may have concerning this procedure will be discussed. For simplicity we will refer to this test as a barium enema.

What Is a Barium Enema?

A **barium enema** is the filling of the large intestine with the radiopaque (seen by X-ray) dye, barium.

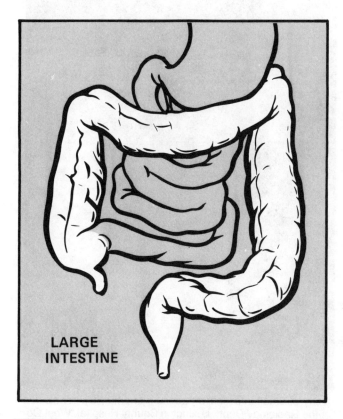

LARGE
INTESTINE

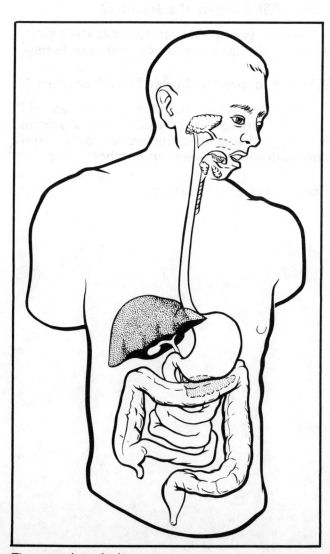

The gastrointestinal system.

Why Is a Barium Enema Done?

A barium enema is done to aid in the diagnosis of tumors, polyps, cancer, and other lesions in the large intestine.

Is There Any Preparation for the Barium Enema?

Yes!
1. If you are going to have this procedure done on an out-patient basis, you will need to go to the X-ray department and pick up instructions and perhaps a kit.
2. The day before the examination you will be given very light meals and asked to drink a glass of water about every hour.
3. The evening meal will consist of clear liquids—no milk, no solids. About ½ hour before the meal, a liquid **cathartic** (medicine to make your bowels move) is given, followed by water.
4. In the evening about 9 o'clock, you are to take 4 pills, also to help your bowels move.
5. The day of your test you will not be given any food until the test is over.

© Robert J. Brady Co., Bowie, MD 20715

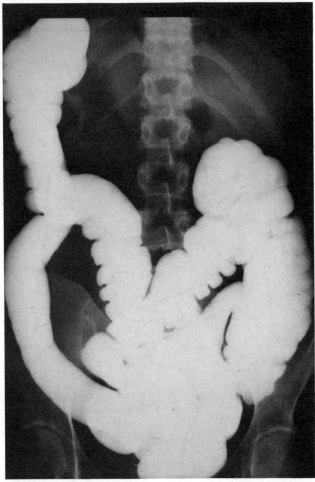

X-ray of small intestine with barium enema. (By permission of the Radiology Dept., Lexington County Hospital, West Columbia, SC.)

6. About an hour before the test, you will be given a small enema to further clean the lower bowel.
7. You will be asked to put on a hospital gown.

Where Will the Test Be Done?

The test will be done in the X-ray department in a special room called a fluoroscopic room.

Who Will Do the Test?

The test will be done by highly trained technologists and a radiologist, who is a specialized physician, using radiation and radioactive materials for medical diagnosis.

How Is the Test Done?

You will be taken to the X-ray department and helped onto a table. You will be made as comfortable as possible. The technologist will ask you to turn on your side. He or she will then insert a lubricated tube into your rectum.

(It will help if you can relax your rectal muscles while the technologist is inserting the tube.) You will now turn onto your back. Now the barium is slowly put through the tube into your rectum. You may feel a crampy sensation during this part of the test. X-ray pictures will now be taken. Try to lie still and retain (hold) the barium in your rectum. The radiologist may put some air into your rectum with a small squeeze bulb. This is called an air-contrast study. This again may cause some cramping. You will then be allowed to expel the enema into a toilet, after which there will be more X-ray pictures taken.

After the procedure, you will be taken back to your room or allowed to leave if your are an outpatient. You will be given time to rest and to eat. It is important that during the first eight hours after the study you drink water or other liquids. This will help to expel the remainder of the barium from your lower bowel.

When Will I Know the Results?

When your physician receives the report, it will be discussed with you and your family.

Will My Insurance Cover This Procedure?

Most health insurance companies will cover the procedure as well as the physician fee. The amount of coverage will differ from one insurance company to another.

Comments and Questions

Your Guide to
Nasogastric Tube Insertion

Introduction

Your doctor has ordered a special test for you called the insertion of a nasogastric tube. We feel it is important that you understand what the test is, why it is being done, and how it is done.

What Is a Nasogastric Tube?

A **nasogastric tube** is a soft rubber or plastic tube that extends from the nose to the stomach.

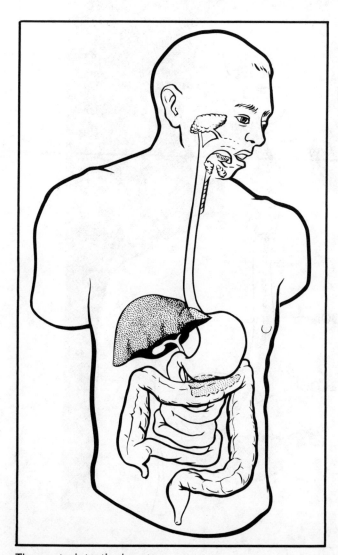

The gastrointestinal system.

Is There Any Preparation for This Test?

You will be asked to put on a hospital gown. The nurse will assist you in getting into a (sitting) position.

Why Is a Nasogastric Tube Inserted?

A nasogastric tube is inserted diagnostically to withdraw contents of the stomach for analysis and to decompress (empty) the stomach. Therapeutically, the nasogastric tube is inserted for iced gastric lavage (washing of the stomach with iced normal saline or salt water), and tube feeding, gastric and intestinal.

Where Is the Test Done?

This test may be done in several areas of the hospital. The most common areas are the patient's bedside, the emergency room, and the operating room.

Who Will Do the Test?

This test may be done by a nurse, technologist, or doctor. All of these members of the health team have been trained to do this procedure.

How Is the Test Done?

You will sit up straight in bed, and be given some tissues. The nurse will hand you a glass of water or ice chips to help you swallow the tube. At this point the nurse will start to insert the lubricated nasogastric tube through your nose. It is not painful, but a little uncomfortable. When you feel the tube in the back of your throat, pant (short breaths) and take sips of the water or ice chips. This action activates the swallowing mechanism. The nurse will slowly insert the tube as you swallow. Your eyes may tear. This is why you were given the tissues. If you cannot have water, try to dry swallow. This will help pass the nasogastric tube. Once the tube is in position, it will be secured to your face with tape.

After the procedure, if the tube was inserted to decompress (empty) the stomach, the tube will be connected to suction. If it is inserted for a feeding tube, it will be clamped

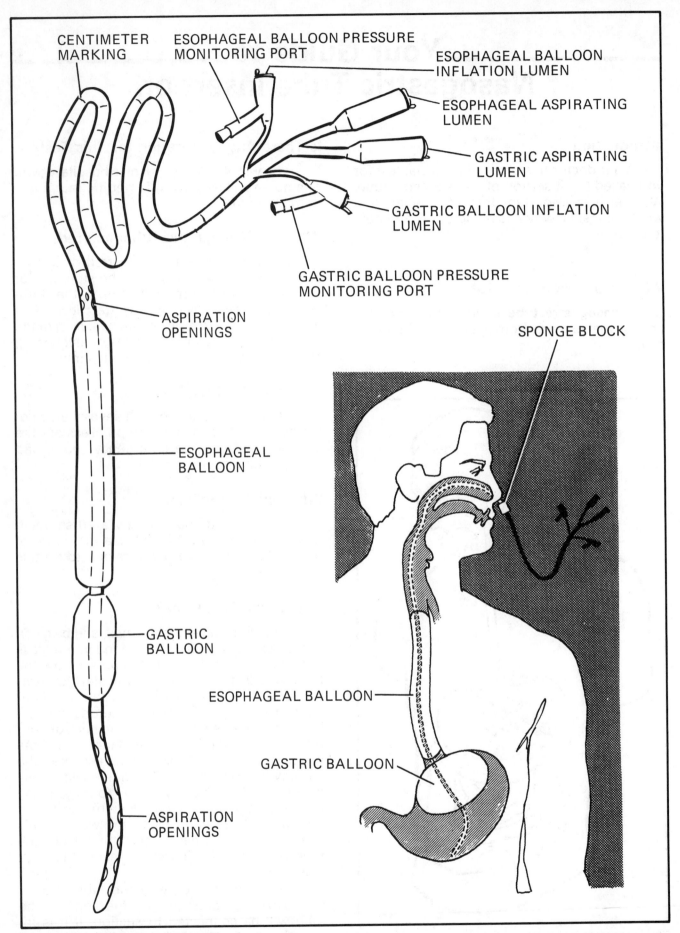

CENTIMETER
MARKING

ESOPHAGEAL BALLOON PRESSURE
MONITORING PORT

ESOPHAGEAL BALLOON
INFLATION LUMEN

ESOPHAGEAL ASPIRATING
LUMEN

GASTRIC ASPIRATING
LUMEN

GASTRIC BALLOON INFLATION
LUMEN

GASTRIC BALLOON PRESSURE
MONITORING PORT

ASPIRATION
OPENINGS

ESOPHAGEAL
BALLOON

GASTRIC
BALLOON

ASPIRATION
OPENINGS

SPONGE BLOCK

ESOPHAGEAL BALLOON

GASTRIC BALLOON

Nasogastric tube diagram and position in stomach.

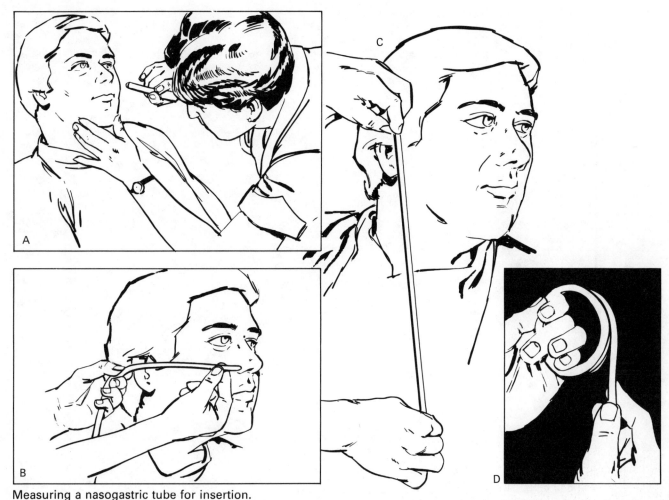

Measuring a nasogastric tube for insertion.

until needed, and secured to the shoulder of your gown.

When Will the Tube Be Removed?

This is a difficult question to answer, because there are so many reasons why the tube is inserted. The average is 3 to 5 days for decompression of the stomach, and up to several weeks for the feeding tube.

Are There Any Complications or Side Effects?

The most common side effects of this procedure are a dry, sore throat and mild discomfort.

Will My Insurance Cover This Procedure?

Most health insurance companies will cover this procedure. The amount of coverage will vary from one company to another.

Comments and Questions

Your Guide to Intestinal Tube Insertion

Introduction

Your doctor has ordered a special test for you called an intestinal tube. We feel it is important that you understand what this procedure is, why the procedure is done, and how the procedure is done. In this information, you will find a discussion of the most frequently asked questions concerning the procedure.

What Is an Intestinal Tube?

An **intestinal tube** is a soft rubber or plastic tube that extends from the nose to the intestine (small bowel).

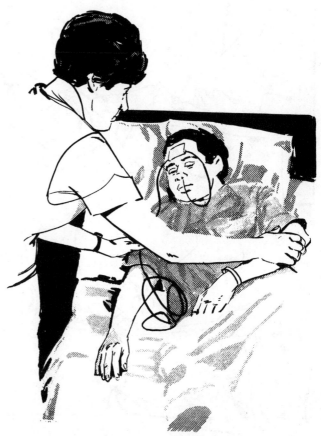
Positioning for intestinal tube placement.

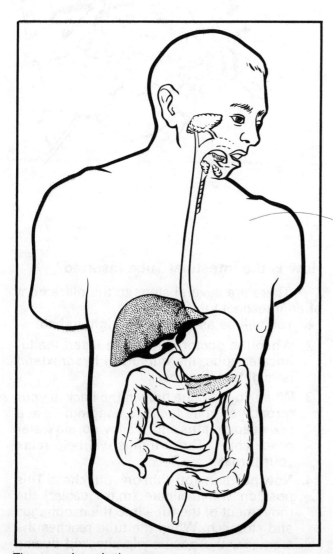
The gastrointestinal system.

Why Is an Intestinal Tube Inserted?

An intestinal tube is inserted for a number of reasons. Diagnostically, the intestinal tube may be inserted to obtain an intestinal contents specimen for analysis. Therapeutically, it is used for relief of bowel obstruction and for intestinal feeding.

What Is the Small Intestine?

The small intestine is a part of the digestive tube extending from the stomach to the junction of the large intestine.

Is There Any Preparation for the Insertion of the Intestinal Tube?

Yes!
1. Water and food will be withheld several hours before the procedure.
2. You will be asked to put on a hospital gown.

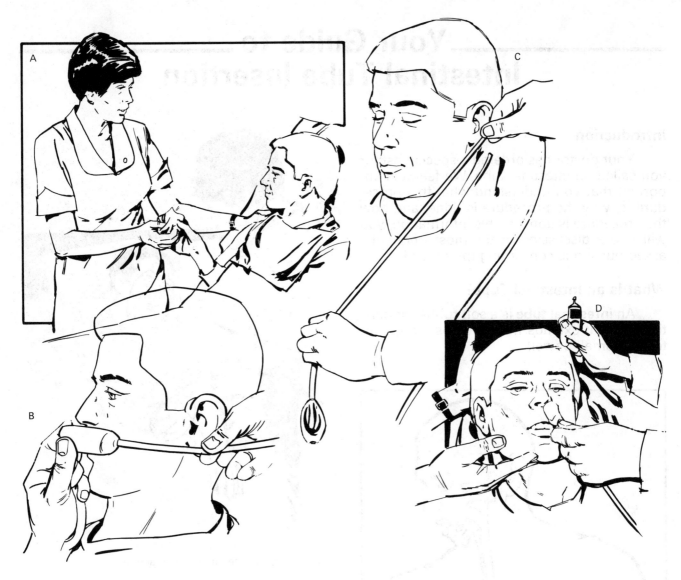

Measuring intestinal tube for insertion.

3. You may be given some medication to help you relax during the procedure.

Is This Procedure Painful?

No! The passage of any tube through your nose is uncomfortable but not painful.

Where Is the Insertion of an Intestinal Tube Done?

The two most common places are the GI laboratory and the patient's bedside.

Who Will Insert the Intestinal Tube?

The intestinal tube is inserted by a physician with the aid of a nurse or technologist.

How Is the Intestinal Tube Inserted?

There are several steps to the placement of an intestinal tube.

1. You will be asked to sit upright in bed.
2. When the doctor is ready to insert the lubricated tube, the nurse will hyperextend (straighten) your neck.
3. When you feel the tube in the back of your throat, you may feel like gagging. Take a few deep breaths and, if allowed, sip water or ice chips. These things will help relax your throat.
4. Now position you chin on your chest. This position will facilitate (make easier) the movement of the tube into the esophagus and stomach. When the tube reaches the stomach, the position is checked by the physician.

5. You will now be asked to turn to your right side. This position facilitates the movement of the tube into your intestine. The location of the tube is checked by aspiration of contents.
6. Every hour the tube is advanced 2 to 3 inches until the correct location is obtained. You will remain on your right side during this time. The location of the tube will be checked by X-ray.

After the procedure, you will be given nose and mouth care often. The tube will be secured to your nose. If there is an abundant amount of tubing left over, it will be secured to the shoulder of your gown by a pin.

When Will the Tube Be Removed?

The doctor will determine when the tube will be removed, based on your physical response to treatment.

Will My Insurance Cover This Procedure?

Most insurance companies will cover this procedure. The amount of coverage will differ from one company to another.

Your Guide to
Gastroscopy

Introduction

Your doctor has ordered a special test for you. It is called a gastroscopy. In this information, you will find a discussion of some of the most frequently asked questions concerning the procedure.

What Is a Gastroscopy?

A **gastroscopy** is a direct examination of the interior of the stomach using a lighted flexible tube.

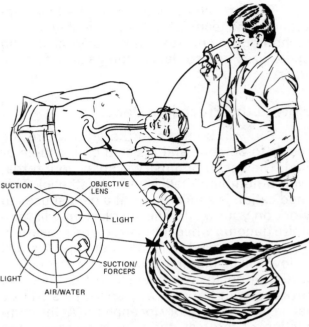

Gastroscope tube inside stomach.

Why Is a Gastroscopy Done?

Diagnostically, a gastroscopy is done for the collection of specimens for the laboratory, and visual examination of the interior of the stomach.

Therapeutically, a gastroscopy is done for the removal of foreign bodies from the gastrointestinal tract.

Is There Any Preparation for This Test?

Yes!
1. Food is withheld at least 6 hours prior to the study.
2. You will be asked to put on a hospital gown.
3. A small needle will be placed in a vein for fluids and/or medication.
4. Medication will be given to help you relax during the procedure.
5. This can be done on an out-patient basis. You must allow at least an hour for the examination and 2 to 3 hours for recovery.
6. If you have dentures, you will be asked to remove them.

Where Is the Procedure Done?

This procedure may be done in a number of localities in the hospital. Some of the more

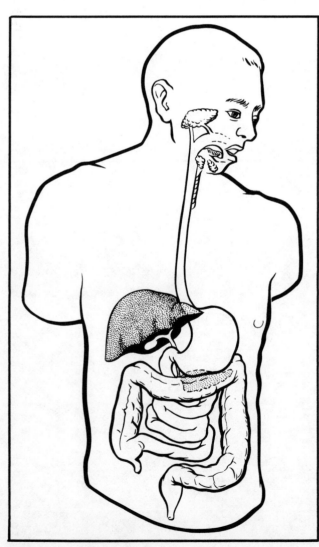

The gastrointestinal system.

common areas are gastrointestinal laboratory, treatment area on general floor, patient's bed side, emergency room, out-patient operating room, etc.

Who Will Do the Procedure?

This procedure is done by the team approach. The team is made up of highly trained technologists, nurses, and a physician who specializes in disorders of the gastrointestinal tract.

How Is the Procedure Done?

You will be taken to the area where the test is to be done and assisted onto a table or bed. The doctor or nurse will spray your throat with a numbing medication (anesthetic). This medication is similar to what a dentist uses to work on your teeth. This medication will minimize gagging when the instrument is inserted. You will be asked to lie on your side. A small pillow will be placed under your head for comfort. The doctor will now insert the tube and proceed with the test. Any specimens will be taken to the laboratory for analysis. At the completion of the test, the tube is removed and you will be made as comfortable as possible.

After the procedure, a nurse will check you frequently. This is the normal routine. You may feel very sleepy from the medication you were given. You will be asked to lie on your side during this period. In about 2 to 3 hours when the gag reflex has returned, you will be allowed to sip on fluids. Hard candy helps to keep your mouth and throat moist.

When Will I Know the Results?

Your physician will discuss the results of the test with you and your family when all of the reports have been received.

Is There Any Complication or Side Effect?

As in any procedure there is always a slight chance of a complication or side effect occurring. However, the diagnostic benefit of having the procedure done far outweighs the risks. A rare complication is gastric perforation. A common side effect is a sore throat.

Will My Insurance Cover This Procedure?

Most health insurance companies will cover the procedure and the physician fee. The amount of coverage will vary from one company to another.

Comments and Questions

© Robert J. Brady Co., Bowie, MD 20715

Your Guide to
Proctoscopy, Sigmoidoscopy
(Proctosigmoidoscopy)

Introduction

Your doctor has ordered a special test for you called a proctosigmoidoscopy. In this information you will find a discussion of the most frequently asked questions concerning this procedure.

What Is a Proctosigmoidscopy?

A **proctoscopy** is the inspection of the anal canal and rectum with a proctoscope. A **sigmoidoscopy** is the inspection of the sigmoid colon (part of the large intestine). A **proctosig-**

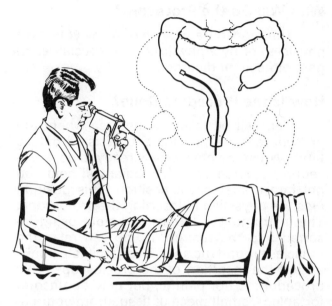

Position of tube in rectum and sigmoid colon.

moidoscopy is the visual inspection of the anal canal, rectum, and the sigmoid colon with a proctoscope.

What Is a Proctoscope?

A **proctoscope** is an instrument for inspecting the anal canal and rectum.

Why Is a Proctosigmoidoscopy Done?

A proctosigmoidoscopy may be done as part of your annual physical after the age of 45. It also may be done to aid in the medical diagnosis of rectal bleeding, hemorrhoids, tumors, constipation, and abdominal pain. During this procedure a **biopsy** (piece of tissue) may be done. A biopsy is simply a piece of tissue taken for examination.

Is There Any Preparation for This Procedure?

Yes!
1. An enema will be given to clear the lower bowel.
2. Food may or may not be withheld, depending upon the doctor's orders.
3. You will be asked to put on a hospital gown.

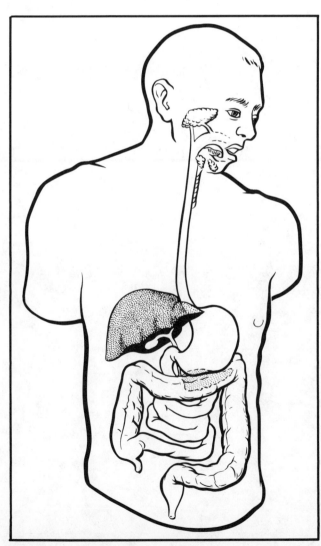

The gastrointestinal system.

Where Is the Procedure Done?

The procedure is usually done in a GE (gastroenterology) department, but may also be done on an out-patient basis in a treatment room, clinic, or physician's office, or at a patient's bedside.

Who Will Do the Procedure?

The procedure may be done by your own physician or by a physician who specializes in gastrointestinal disorders.

How Is the Procedure Done?

You will be taken to the area where the procedure is to be done and assisted onto a table. When the physician is ready to do a procedure, a nurse or technologist will help you get into a knee-chest position. This position aids the physician in inserting the protoscope. The instrument is lubricated before being inserted into the rectum. If you can relax the muscles around the anus, it will facilitate (make easier) the insertion of the proctoscope. This procedure is not painful, but may be uncomfortable. A small piece of tissue from your colon may be taken and sent to the laboratory for analysis. This is called a biopsy. It is not painful to have a biopsy done.

Are There Any Complicatons or Side Effects?

1. If a biopsy was obtained, there may be a small amount of blood in the stool.
2. If air was introduced during the study, you may have some cramping during the test and pass some flatus (gas) post test.

When Will I Know the Results of the Test?

The physician will tell you of the results of the proctosigmoidoscopy procedures as soon as all the information from the test is known.

Will My Insurance Cover This Procedure?

Most health insurance companies will cover the procedure and the physician fee. The amount of coverage will vary from one insurance company to another.

Comments and Questions

Your Guide to Oral Cholecystography

Introduction

Your doctor has ordered a special X-ray procedure of your gallbladder called an oral cholecystogram. In this information, there will be a discussion of the most frequently asked questions concerning this procedure.

What Is an Oral Cholecystogram?

An **oral cholecystogram** is a radiograph (X-ray picture) of the gallbladder.

What Is a Cholecystography?

A cholecystography is an X-ray picture of the gallbladder after the ingestion (swallowing

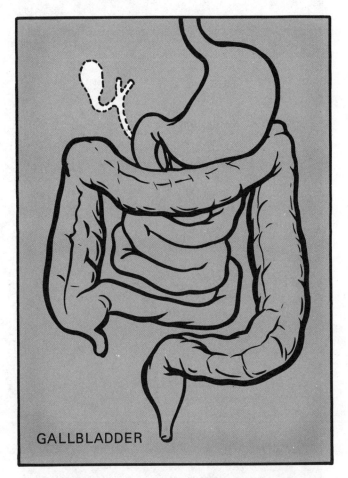

GALLBLADDER

liquid or pills) or intravenous injection of a radiopaque (seen by X-ray) substance excreted in the bile.

Is There Any Special Preparation for This Procedure?

Yes!
1. You will be asked if you are allergic to iodine or shellfish. The dye used in this procedure contains iodine.
2. You will have low-fat meals the day before the test.
3. After your dinner you will be given 6 or more dye tablets to take with a full (8 oz.) glass of water.
4. After you drink this water, do not eat or drink anything until the procedure is over.
5. You will be asked to put on a hospital gown.
6. This procedure may be done on an outpatient basis.

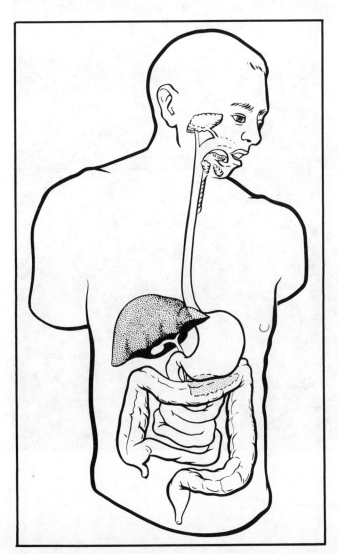

The gastrointestinal system.

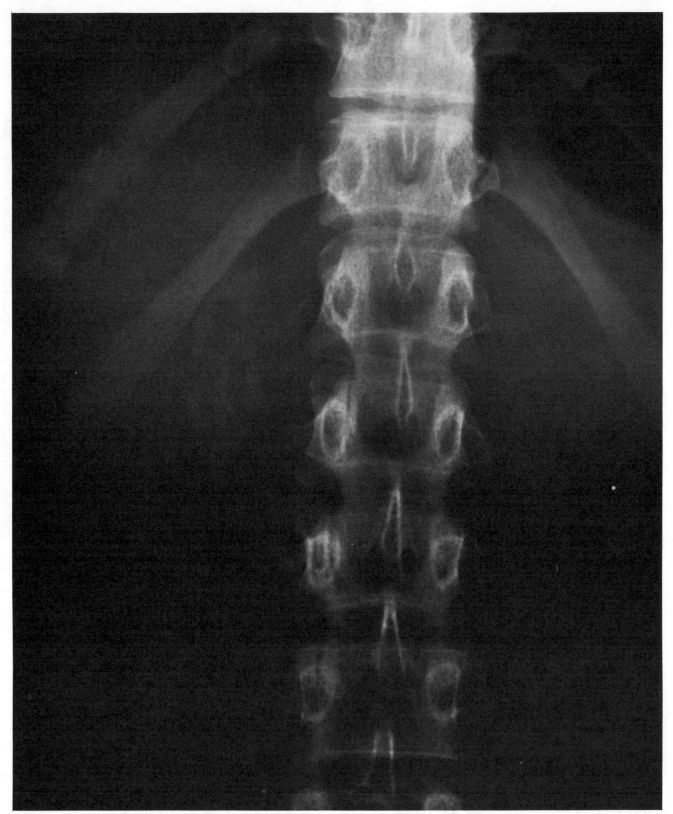

Cholecystogram of gallbladder with stones. (By permission
of the Diagnostic Radiology Clinic, Columbia, SC, Sarah M.
Klein, MD, Radiologist.)

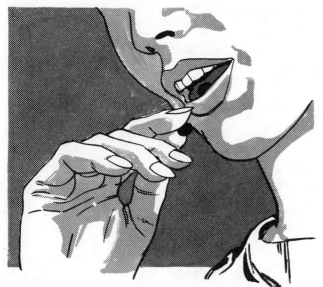

Taking dye tablets.

Will My Insurance Cover This Procedure?

Most health insurance companies will cover the procedure and the physician fee. The amount of coverage will differ from one company to another.

Comments and Questions

Where Is the Cholecystogram Procedure Done?

The cholecystogram procedure is done in the radiology (X-ray) department.

Who Will Do the Cholecystogram Procedure?

The cholecystogram procedure is done by highly trained technologists and a radiologist. A **radiologist** is a physician who specializes in the use of radiation and radioactive materials for medical diagnosis.

How Is the Cholecystogram Done?

You will be taken to the X-ray department and assisted onto the table. X-ray pictures will be taken of your gallbladder, and you will be returned to your room or if you are an outpatient, you may return home.

When Will I Know the Results?

When your physician receives the report from X-ray, it will be discussed with you and your family.

Are There Any Complications or Side Effects?

Side effects in this procedure are rare. If you are sensitive to the tablets, you may break out in a rash, become nauseated, or vomit.

Your Guide to
IV and T-Tube Cholangiography

Introduction

Your doctor has ordered a special X-ray study of the bile ducts of your gallbladder. These tests are done after you have had your gallbladder removed by surgery. In this information you will find a discussion of the most frequently asked questions concerning these procedures.

What Is an IV Cholangiogram?

An **IV cholangiogram** is an X-ray picture of the bile ducts of the gallbladder after the injection of an intravenous contrast medium (dye).

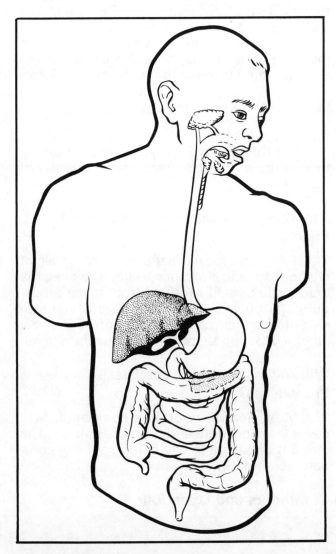

The gastrointestinal system.

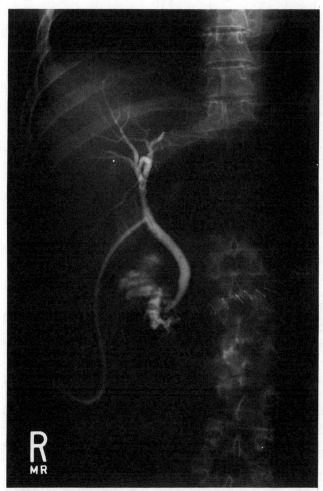

T-tube cholangiogram. (By permission of the Radiology Dept., Richland Memorial Hospital, Cola, SC.)

Why Is an IV Cholangiogram Done?

An IV cholangiogram is done if the patient has recurring symptoms after the gallbladder has been surgically removed.

What Is a T-Tube Cholangiogram?

A **T-tube cholangiogram** is an X-ray picture of the common bile ducts of the gallbladder after injection of dye into the T-tube drain.

Why Is a T-Tube Cholangiogram Done?

A T-tube cholangiogram is done to determine if the common bile duct is open before the T-tube drain is removed.

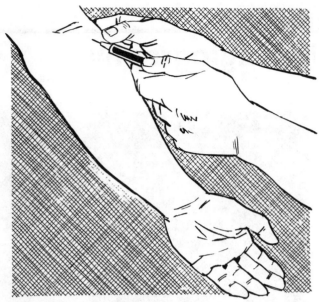
Injecting dye into a vein.

Is There Any Preparation for These Procedures?

Yes!

1. It is very important that the doctor knows if you are allergic to iodine or shellfish. A large portion of the dye is iodine.
2. A low-fat meal is given the evening before the study and then *do not* eat or drink anything until the test is over. This is called NPO (nothing by mouth).
3. You will be asked to put on a hospital gown the morning of the study.
4. If you do not have a capped intravenous needle or an IV, one will be started. A nurse

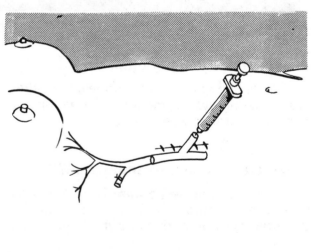
Injecting dye into a t-tube.

will put a small needle in your vein for fluids and/or medications.

5. The doctor may order preoperative medication to help you relax if you are having a T-tube cholangiogram.

Where Will These Procedures Be Done?

Both of these studies are radiographic (X-ray procedures) and thus will be done in the X-ray department.

Who Will Do These Procedures?

These procedures will be done by highly trained technologists and a radiologist. A **radiologist** is a physician who specializes in the use of radiation and radioactive materials for medical diagnosis.

How Are These Procedures Done?

An intravenous cholangiogram is done by the injection of dye into a vein. Then an X-ray picture is taken of the bile ducts.

A T-tube cholangiogram is done by the injection of dye through the T-tube. X-ray pictures are then taken of the common bile ducts.

When Will I Know the Results of the Tests?

Your doctor will tell you and your family the results of the test when they are received from X-ray.

Are There Any Complications or Side Effects?

As in any procedure there is always a slight chance of a side effect occurring. However, the diagnostic benefit received from these procedures far outweighs the risk. Two of the rare side effects that may occur are infection or an allergic reaction to the contrast medium (dye).

Will My Insurance Cover These Procedures?

Most health insurance companies will cover the procedure and the physician fee. The amount of coverage will differ from one company to another.

Comments and Questions

Your Guide to
Abdominal Paracentesis

Introduction

Your doctor has ordered a special test (procedure) for you called paracentesis. In this information, you will find a discussion of the most frequently asked questions concerning the procedure.

What Is Abdominal Paracentesis?

Abdominal paracentesis is a puncture of the abdominal cavity by means of a hollow needle.

Why Is Abdominal Paracentesis Done?

Abdominal paracentesis is done diagnostically to determine intra-abdominal bleeding from injury, and for the laboratory analysis of abdominal fluid or ascitic fluid. Therapeutically, abdominal paracentesis may be done to relieve urinary frequency due to pressure, or to relieve dyspnea (difficult breathing).

Is There Any Special Preparation for This Procedure?

Yes!
1. You should try to void or urinate (pass water) before the procedure.
2. You will be asked to put on a hospital gown for the procedure.
3. Food will be withheld for several hours before the procedure.
4. A small needle will be inserted into your vein for fluids and/or medication.
5. You may be given some medication to help you relax during the procedure.

Where Is the Paracentesis Done?

The paracentesis may be done in a treatment room, emergency room, operating room, or at the patient's bedside. Other areas of the hospital may be used, but the emergency room and the patient's bedside are the two most common areas.

Who Will Do the Paracentesis?

The paracentesis will be done by a physician and a nurse or technologist who have been trained in the procedure.

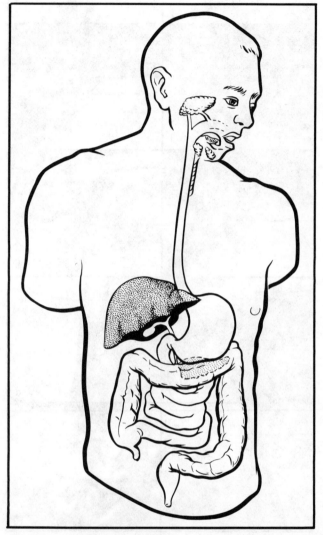

The gastrointestinal system.

How Is the Procedure Done?

You will be asked to sit up in a chair or in a high Fowler's position (sitting) in bed. The physician will then clean the abdomen with an antiseptic (germ-killing) solution and establish a sterile (germ-free) field with sterile towels. It is very important that you *do not touch* these sterile towels. The physician will now inject the area with an anesthetic (numbing medication). This is very much like the medication the dentist uses to work on your teeth. The next step is to make a small incision in the abdomen, followed by the insertion of a specialized nee-

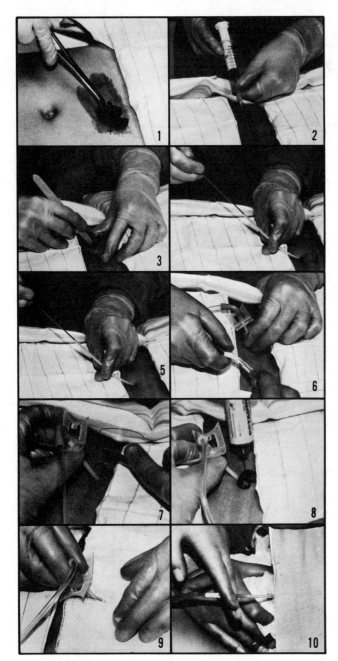

Inserting needle for abdominal paracentesis.

When Will I Know the Results of the Test?

Your doctor will tell you and your family the results of the laboratory analysis as soon as possible.

Are There Any Complications or Side Effects?

As in any procedure, there is always a slight chance of a complication or side effect occurring. However, the diagnostic and/or therapeutic benefits gained from the procedure far outweigh the risk! A few *rare* complications are a drop in blood pressure due to rapid withdrawal of fluid, puncture of bowel or other organ, and infection.

Will My Insurance Cover This Procedure?

Most insurance companies will cover the procedure as well as the physician's fee. The amount of coverage will vary from one company to another.

Comments and Questions

dle called a **trocar**. The doctor will remove the metal guide of the needle and a plastic cannula (tube) is left in place. The doctor will allow a specific amount of fluid to drain from the abdomen. This fluid is then sent to the laboratory for analysis. The cannula is removed and a dry, sterile dressing is applied.

After the procedure, you will be returned to your room. A nurse will check your vital signs frequently. This is a normal procedure. At this time, the nurse will also check your dressing.

Your Guide to Percutaneous Liver Biopsy

Introduction

Your doctor has ordered a special test for you. It is called a percutaneous liver biopsy. We want you to understand what a liver biopsy is, why, and how it is done. In this information, you will find a discussion of some of the most frequently asked questions concerning the procedure.

What Is a Percutaneous Liver Biopsy?

Let us define this each word at a time. **Percutaneous**—through the skin; **Liver**—an organ located in the abdomen; **Biopsy**—the

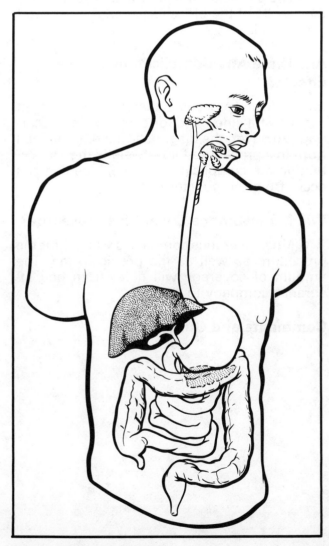

The gastrointestinal system.

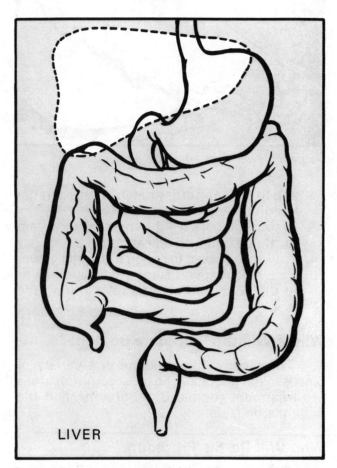

Dashed line shows position of liver.

excision (cutting) of a piece of body tissue for diagnostic study. Combining these definitions, you have an excision of a piece of liver tissue by entry through the skin.

Why Is a Percutaneous Liver Biopsy Done?

A percutaneous liver biopsy is done to confirm diagnosis of cirrhosis or cancer of the liver.

Is There Any Preparation for This Procedure?

Yes!
1. Food will be withheld for about 6 hours before the procedure and until the procedure is over.
2. A blood sample will be drawn prior to the test to assess the coagulation (clotting) time,

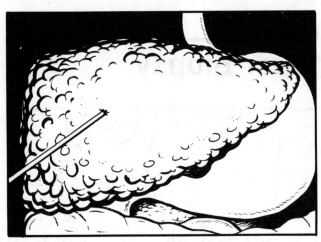
Diagram of liver showing needle position.

and to type and crossmatch in case a transfusion is needed.
3. A small needle will be inserted in a vein for fluids and/or medication.
4. You will be asked to put on a hospital gown.
5. You will be given some medication prior to the study to help you relax during the test.

Where Will the Procedure Be Done?

The biopsy may be done in a variety of places in the hospital. The most common areas are treatment rooms, GI laboratory, and the patient's bedside.

Who Will Do the Procedure?

The procedure will be done utilizing the team approach. The team is composed of a nurse, laboratory or GI technologist, and a physician. All of these team members are trained in the biopsy procedure.

Will the Procedure Hurt?

You may feel pressure, but should not feel pain. The premedication will also help you relax.

How Is the Procedure Done?

You will be taken to the area where the procedure is to be done. A nurse or another member of the health team will assist you onto a table where you will be positioned on your left side. Your right side will be exposed and a pillow placed under your head and right shoulder. The doctor will scrub the area with an antiseptic (germ-killing) solution and establish a sterile (germ-free) field with sterile towels. It is very important that you *do not touch*

this area. Then the area is injected with a numbing medication (anesthetic). This is much like the medication the dentist uses when working on your teeth. The physician will now insert a special needle into your liver. You will be asked to hold your breath during this time (only about 5 to 10 seconds). The biopsy (liver tissue sample) is taken and the needle is removed.

After the procedure, a pressure dressing is applied to the puncture site and you will be returned to your room. You will be instructed to lie on your right side for 2 hours to splint the puncture site. You are *not* to get out of bed for 24 hours after the procedure. This is called complete bed rest. It *does not* mean that you can get up and go to the bathroom. During this period of time, you will use a bedpan and/or urinal.

When Will I Know the Results?

The physician will tell you and your family the results of the biopsy as soon as the report is received.

Are There Any Complication or Side Effects?

As in any procedure, there is always a slight chance of a side effect or complication occurring. However, the diagnostic benefit obtained from this procedure far outweighs the risk. Although the complication is rare, bleeding can occur from the puncture site.

Will My Insurance Cover This Procedure?

Most insurance companies will pay for the procedure as well as the physician fee. The amount of coverage will differ from one insurance company to another.

Comments and Questions

6
Urologic Procedures

Urine Collection

There is a variety of methods of obtaining a urine specimen for diagnostic laboratory analysis. A few of these methods are: (1) clean catch specimen (obtained by voiding into a urine specimen cup after thoroughly cleaning the area around the urethra); (2) midstream specimen (obtained by cleaning urethral opening, starting stream, stopping and then restarting stream and collecting specimen); (3) catheterized specimen (entering the bladder of the patient via the urethra utilizing a catheter, and done under sterile technique; and (4) 24-hour urine (urinary specimen collected for 24 hours to obtain qualitative and quantitative analysis of specific urinary by-products).

Nurse's Responsibilities

Pre-Test
1. Explain the procedure to the patient and family (may be done as out-patient).
2. Supply patient with necessary specimen cups, wipes, etc.
3. Provide privacy for patient.

Precautions
1. Instruct patient in proper way to clean urethra opening.
2. Instruct patient in the importance of not contaminating specimen cup.
3. During 24-hour urine, emphasize the importance of collecting *all* of the urine and any special directions; i.e., ice, acid, etc.

Post-Procedure
1. Send collected urine specimen to laboratory for analysis. Ensure specimen is properly marked.
2. If procedure is done as an out-patient, instruct patient where to take specimen.

Urethral Catheterization

Urethral catheterization may be done for diagnostic as well as therapeutic reasons. Diagnostically, urethral catheterization is done to obtain a urine specimen for laboratory analysis. Therapeutically, urethral catheterization may be done to relieve urinary frequency, pressure, empty the bladder, and instill medication into the bladder.

This procedure is indicated in patients who have or are suspected of having infections of the urinary system, post-urologic surgery, trauma, inability to void, urinary calculi, urinary frequency, inflammatory disorder, functional disorder, and others.

Nurse's Responsibilities

Pre-Test
1. Explain the procedure to the patient and family.
2. No dietary preparation.
3. Have patient put on a hospital gown.
4. Ensure privacy for the patient during the procedure. Explain to the patient that you will protect his or her privacy as much as possible.
5. Inform the patient that you will need his or her cooperation.
6. Inform the patient that slow deep breathing and muscle relaxation will ensure an easy and pain-free entry into the bladder.

Precautions
1. If bleeding begins with insertion of the catheter, withdraw the catheter and call physician.
2. If catheter cannot be advanced into bladder, try a smaller French-size catheter. If it still cannot be advanced, withdraw catheter and inform physician.
3. Never withdraw more than 700–800 ml at one time. Either clamp the catheter or withdraw it. Reinsert catheter at the physician's request.
4. Do not leave urinary specimens on the floor for any length of time. Send them to the laboratory as soon as possible.
5. It is essential for patient that urethral catheterization is done as a sterile procedure. Self-catheterization utilizing clean technique is not pertinent to this procedure.

Post-Procedure
1. Assist patient in cleaning up after procedure.
2. Allow patient time to rest after procedure.
3. If catheter is left in the patient, secure the tubing to the woman's leg or man's abdomen and attach the catheter to the appropriate drainage system.

Intravenous Pyelography (IVP)

An IVP is an X-ray of the renal system utilizing intravenous contrast media or dye. It is one of the most frequent renal procedures done in the radiology department.

This procedure is indicated in patients who have or are suspected of having urinary obstruction of varied etiologies or to assess kidney function.

Nurse's Responsibilities

Pre-Test
1. Explain the procedure to the patient and family (may be done as an out-patient).
2. Ask patient if he or she is allergic to iodine or shellfish.
3. A laxative is usually given to clear out the intestinal system for greater visualization of the urological system.
4. Patient will be NPO post midnight until after the procedure.
5. In some hospitals a permit may be necessary. If one has not been signed, ask the patient to sign one and witness his or her signature.
6. Help patient into a hospital gown.
7. Have patient void prior to procedure.
8. Explain to the patient that he or she may feel some burning when the dye is injected. It will only last a short time.
9. Have patient and chart ready for transfer to Radiology Department.

Precautions
1. This procedure is contraindicated for the patient who is allergic to shellfish or iodine.
2. Patient should be cooperative and able to follow orders.
3. The procedure area should be equipped with emergency equipment and drugs.

Post-Procedure
1. Monitor vital signs as per order.
2. When all X-rays are done, patient may eat.
3. Fluids should be encouraged—dye is excreted through the kidneys.
4. Keep an accurate intake and output record.
5. Inform physician if patient has not voided in 6 to 8 hours.
6. Inform physician if patient has a delayed reaction to dye (difficulty in breathing, urticaria, etc.).

Cytoscopy or Panendoscopy

A cytoscopy is the internal inspection of the uretha and bladder utilizing a cystoscope. This procedure may be done under local or general anesthesia. It is done to assess urinary tract disorders.

Nurse's Responsibilities

Pre-Test
1. Explain procedure to patient and family (may be done as an out-patient). Patient may be anxious. Allow him or her to verbalize fears, then reassure patient.
2. If a permit has not been obtained, get one signed and witnessed.
3. If general anesthesia is to be used, instruct patient not to eat or drink anything 8 hours prior to procedure.
4. Have patient put on a hospital gown.
5. Have patient void prior to procedure.
6. Explain to patient that he or she may have some burning on urination after procedure.
7. Have patient and chart ready for transfer to procedure area.
8. Give pre-medication on call as per order.

Precautions
1. This procedure is contraindicated in acute infections of the bladder, urethra, or prostate gland.
2. If procedure is to be done under local, the patient should know in order to cooperate.

Post-Procedure
1. Monitor vital signs as per order. If patient had general anesthesia, he or she may go to recovery room for reaction.
2. Keep an accurate intake and output.
3. Encourage patient to drink fluids.
4. Ensure patient that a small amount of blood and burning on urination are normal post procedure.
5. Inform physician if frank bleeding, abdominal pain, chills, anuria, flank pain or fever develops.
6. Administer analgesics and antibiotics as per order post procedure.

Urethrography and Cystourethrography

A urethrography is a radiographic examination of the urethra after the injection or instillation of an opaque contrast media. A cystourethrography is a radiographic examination of the bladder and urethra after the injection of a contrast media.

A urethrographic examination is done to visualize abnormalities of the urethra (strictures, obstructions, lacerations, trauma, or congenital abnormalities). A cystourethrographic examination is done to visualize abnormalities of the bladder or the urethra (functional and anatomic abnormalities of the bladder, physiological integrity of the bladder, as well as urethral abnormalities delineated above). In a voiding cystourethrography, contrast media is instilled into the bladder and radiographic films are taken of the patient voiding. This radiographic examination is indicated in patients with chronic urinary infections, incontinence, congenital abnormalities, and inability to empty bladder completely.

Nurse's Responsibilities

Pre-Test
1. Explain procedure to patient and family (may be done on an out-patient basis).

2. Obtain a written permit if one has not been already obtained.
3. Reassure the patient that his or her privacy will be safeguarded as much as possible.
4. Inform the patient that the procedure is not painful but may be uncomfortable.
5. Food is usually not restricted prior to the study.
6. Have patient put on a hospital gown.
7. Have patient void prior to the procedure.
8. Check the chart for hypersensitivity to contrast media or iodine.
9. Have patient and chart ready for transfer to radiology department.
10. Administer pre-medication as per order on call for the procedure.

Precautions
1. Any of these procedures should be performed with utmost care in patients with urinary tract infections.
2. Recent barium studies may obstruct the view.
3. These are safer procedures for patients allergic to iodine than those procedures that utilize the intravenous route for contrast media. Physician and radiologist need to be aware if the patient is hypersensitive to iodinated products.
4. Procedure area should have emergency equipment and medications available.

Post-Procedure
1. Make patient comfortable, allow patient time to rest.
2. Keep strict I&O record.
3. Note time, amount, and color of first voiding.
4. Reassure patient that some soreness and burning on urination is normal.
5. Encourage fluid intake.
6. Observe patient for fever or chills, which might denote sepsis.
7. If hematuria continues post second to third voiding, notify physician.
8. Observe for post procedure hypersensitivity reaction to contrast media.

Cystography and Retrograde Pyleography

Cystography and retrograde pyleography are radiographic and urologic procedures utilizing contrast media injected through a cystoscope. These procedures allow for visualization of the kidneys, ureters, and bladder. Cystography is done to assess bladder function and to detect the presence of tumors, polyps, or stones in the bladder. Retrograde pyleography is done to assess the anatomical structure of the kidneys (calyces, renal pelvis) and ureters as well as to detect congenital abnormalities, calculi, strictures, and other obstructions of the renal collecting system.

It is important to note that this is a fairly safe procedure for those patients who are allergic to contrast media. It is also important to note that this procedure may be done safely in patients with renal insufficiency.

Nurse's Responsibilities

Pre-Test
1. Explain the procedure to the patient and family (may be done as an out-patient).
2. Obtain a written permit if one has not already been obtained.
3. This procedure may be done utilizing local or general anesthesia.
4. Patients are usually anxious. Let them verbalize their fears, then reassure them.
5. If general anesthesia is to be given, the patient should be NPO 8 hours prior to the study.
6. If a local anesthesia is to be used, explain to the patient that there may be some discomfort and pressure throughout the procedure.
7. Bowel (large) prep may be done to remove fecal material.
8. Many physicians request that their patients have an IV placed prior to the start of the study.
9. Have patient put on a hospital gown.
10. If general anesthesia is to be used, have patient remove dentures or bridges.
11. Have patient void prior to the procedure.
12. Have patient and chart ready for transfer to procedure area.
13. Give pre-medication on call as per order.

Precautions
1. Caution should be used in doing this procedure on a patient with known ureteral obstruction.
2. Fecal material in large intestine may obstruct view.
3. Barium from previous studies may obstruct view.
4. Procedure area should be equipped with emergency equipment and medications.

Post-Procedure
1. If patient had general anesthesia, he or she may go to recovery room for reaction.
2. Monitor vital signs as per order.
3. Encourage fluid intake.
4. Note amount, time, color of first voiding.
5. If patient has not voided 8 hours post-procedure, notify physician.
6. Keep an accurate I&O record.
7. Notify physician if patient continues to have hematuria past the second or third voiding or if it is a large amount.
8. Reassure patient that discomfort and burning on urination is normal post procedure.
9. Observe patient for severe pain in kidney region, chills, fever, or other signs of sepsis or perforation. Notify physician immediately.
10. If ureteral catheters or a foley catheter has been left in place, secure to patient's leg and note drainage.
11. Administer analgesics as per order for discomfort.

Cystometrography

Cystometrography is a graphic assessment of the neuromuscular function of the bladder. This test measures the efficiency of the detrusor muscle, the intravesical pressure and capacity of the bladder, as well as the bladder's reaction to hot and cold stimuli. The purpose of this procedure is to determine the cause of a neurogenic bladder, to evaluate bladder muscle tonicity, to assess detrusor muscle function, and to aid in the diagnosis of bladder dysfunction.

Nurse's Responsibilities

Pre-Test
1. Explain procedure to the patient and family (may be done as an out-patient).
2. Check chart for permit. If one has not been obtained, have one signed and witnessed.
3. Inform patient that the procedure is not painful but may be uncomfortable.
4. Inform the patient that there may be times when the test is embarrassing.
5. Food or fluids are usually not restricted.
6. Have patient put on a hospital gown.
7. Important to note any medications that may affect the results of the procedure. Notify physician.
8. Have patient and chart ready for transfer to procedure area.

Precautions
1. It is very important that the *full* cooperation of the patient is obtained.
2. Erroneous results can be obtained due to embarrassment if the patient is not well prepared.
3. This procedure, like most of the other urologic procedures, should not be done on a patient with an acute urinary tract infection.
4. Test results may be misleading if medications are taken concurrently that can interfere with the procedure (antihistamines, muscle relaxants).
5. Straining can cause misleading results.
6. Patients who have had spinal cord surgery due to injuries, neoplasms, etc., *should not* be studied until 2 to 3 months post surgery.
7. Patients with muscular diseases (multiple sclerosis, muscular dystrophy, etc.) or spinal cord injury should be transported by stretcher. The test can be done on the stretcher without transporting the patient to a table.

Post-Procedure
1. Make patient comfortable and allow time for patient to relax.
2. Assure patient that burning and discomfort on urination is normal post procedure.
3. Keep an accurate I&O record.
4. Note time, color, and amount of first voiding.
5. If hematuria persists, notify physician.

6. Observe patient for signs of sepsis (fever, chills, discomfort). Notify physician.
7. A warm bath may help discomfort.
8. Administer analgesics as per order for discomfort.

Renal Biopsy and Percutaneous Aspiration

A percutaneous renal biopsy is the excision of kidney tissue utilizing a hollow needle. The specimen is sent for laboratory analysis. This procedure is done less often today since the advent of renal ultrasonography and computerized axial tomography.

Its purpose is to aid in the diagnosis of renal parenchymal disease, tumors (benign and metastatic), and cysts, and to follow the progression of renal disease. This procedure is also helpful in the evaluation of therapeutic treatment of renal disease.

Nurse's Responsibilities

Pre-Test
1. Explain the procedure to the patient and family.
2. Obtain a written permit.
3. Patient will be NPO 8 hours prior to procedure.
4. Check chart for appropriate blood work including coagulation studies.
5. Check chart for hypersensitivity to local anesthetics.
6. Inform patient that the test will be done under a local anesthetic and that it will sting.
7. Check IV for infiltration. If patient does not have an IV, start one with an 18g or larger needle.
8. Inform the patient that he or she will feel pressure and possibly pinching pain as the needle penetrates the kidney.
9. Have patient put on a hospital gown.
10. Have patient void prior to the procedure.
11. Have patient and chart ready for transport to procedure area. (May be done in the radiology department.)
12. Administer pre-medication on call for the procedure.

Precautions
1. This procedure is contraindicated in a number of renal disease processes (renal solid tumor, hydronephrosis, *only one kidney*, renal failure, or renal abscess).
2. This procedure is also contraindicated in severe systematic hypertension, bleeding disorder, or decreased blood volume.
3. When biopsy is obtained, label it correctly and send it to the laboratory for analysis.
4. Patient should be cooperative and able to follow directions.

Post-Procedure
1. Make patient comfortable.
2. Monitor vital signs as per order: q15 min X4, q30 min X4, q1 hr X4, q4 hr.
3. Observe puncture site for drainage.
4. Encourage fluid intake.
5. Inform patient that he or she should be on strict bed rest for 8 hours post procedure.
6. Patient may resume his or her normal diet.
7. Keep an accurate I&O record.
8. Note time, amount, and color of first urine voided.
9. Notify physician if an unusual amount of hematuria is present.
10. Notify physician of flank pain, abdominal pain, fever, chills, change in vital signs that may denote hemorrhage, sepsis, or perforation.
11. Administer analgesics as per order for discomfort.

Peritoneal Dialysis

Peritoneal dialysis is the diffusion of solute molecules through a semipermeable membrane (peritoneum). These solute molecules pass from a higher concentration through the membrane to a lower concentration. This procedure is indicated in individuals with renal failure. The renal failure may be temporary or permanent. The purpose of the procedure is: (1) to maintain adequate clearance of metabolites from the blood; (2) to assist in the regulation of fluid and electrolyte balance; (3) to remove excessive body fluid; and (4) to assist in the maintenance of blood pressure until renal function is restored or the decision to continue with peritoneal or hemodialysis is made.

Nurse's Responsibilities

Pre-Test
1. Reinforce the explanation of the procedure given by the physician to the patient and family.
2. Ensure that a written permit has been obtained.
3. Give the patient and family time to ventilate their feelings and fears.
4. Gather all necessary equipment and medications needed for the procedure.
5. If physician is going to insert the peritoneal catheter, you will need a peritoneal tray and catheter.
6. Check chart for hypersensitivity to anesthestic agents.
7. Explain the procedure for placement of the catheter to patient.
8. Have patient put on a hospital gown.
9. Have patient void.
10. Position patient on his or her back.
11. Administer analgesics or sedative as per order.
12. Assist physician with insertion of peritoneal catheter.

13. Take patient's vital signs and note what patient's weight was in morning.
14. Check central or peripheral IV line for patency and signs of infiltration.
15. Begin peritoneal dialysis according to physician orders and hospital procedure.

Precautions
1. Important that patient is on a high protein diet to make up for protein loss.
2. Bleeding tendency is a contraindication for this procedure.
3. Leakage around the peritoneal dialysis catheter predisposes the patient to the most common complication of dialysis—peritonitis.
4. If patient experiences pain on infusion of the fluid, it may be due to improper temperature of the fluid.
5. Withdrawing large amounts of peritoneal fluid too quickly may lead to shock!
6. If patient experiences respiratory difficulty, it may be due to the amount of fluid in the peritoneal cavity. The fluid may create upward displacement of the diaphragm.

Post-Procedure
1. Cover dialysis tube with a cap.
2. Clean area around tube and apply dry sterile dressing.
3. Make patient comfortable and give him or her time to rest.
4. Monitor patient's vital signs as per order.
5. Keep an accurate I&O record.
6. Observe patient for signs of peritonitis, bleeding, or hypovolemic shock. Notify physician immediately.
7. Administer analgesics as per order for discomfort.

Insertion of an Arteriovenous (A-V) Shunt, Fistula, or Graft

One of these procedures will be done in preparation for hemodialysis. An A-V shunt is an anastomosis between an artery and vein by surgical means. An A-V fistula is an abnormal pathway between two surfaces (artery-vein), and an A-V graft is an anastomosis utilizing a man-made or bovine graft between an artery and vein. The procedure performed will depend upon the physician's choice and the length of time the patient will need dialysis.

Nurse's Responsibilities

Pre-Test
1. Explain the procedure to the patient and family.
2. Obtain a written permit if one has not been obtained.
3. Patient will be NPO for 8 hours prior to procedure.
4. Have patient put on a hospital gown.
5. Have patient void prior to procedure.

6. Have patient remove dentures or loose bridges.
7. Ensure patient and chart are ready for transfer to the operating room.
8. Give pre-medication as per order on call for procedure.

Precautions

1. These procedures are contraindicated in a patient in septic shock or acute septicemia.
2. All of these procedures run the risk of infection and blood clots.
3. An A-V fistula cannot be done in a patient with very small veins.
4. Diabetic patients who have an A-V fistula or graft run the risk of developing steal syndrome.
5. Never draw blood or take blood pressure in the extremity with a shunt, fistula, or graft.

Post-Procedure

1. Monitor vital signs as per order.
2. Make patient comfortable—elevate the limb with the shunt, fistula, or graft.
3. Check dressing for drainage and/or infection.
4. Ask patient to stay in bed for 24 hours post procedure.
5. Monitor site for good arterial flow and any abnormal bruit or thrill.
6. Have clamps available at bedside in case of bleeding. Notify physician immediately.
7. Post a sign over patient's bed—"No blood drawing or blood pressure from shunt, fistula, or graft site." Inform patient not to wear constrictive clothing.

Hemodialysis

Hemodialysis is the process of cleaning the blood of metabolic waste products and removing excess fluid utilizing a concentration gradient and semi-permeable membrane. It is indicated for patients who are in acute renal failure.

Nurse's Responsibilities

Pre-Test

1. Explain procedure to patient and family or reinforce what physician has said.
2. Ensure a written permit has been obtained.
3. Have patient eat an early breakfast if patient is to be taken to dialysis early in the morning.
4. Weigh patient and obtain vital signs.
5. Check medication orders to see if patient will need any medication while in dialysis.
6. Observe shunt, fistula, or graft site for any signs of infection, inflammation, or blood clot.
7. Have patient and chart ready for transport to dialysis unit.

Precautions

1. Sterile technique must be used to ensure freedom from infection.
2. Patient must be monitored closely to prevent a rapid decrease in blood pressure. (A 10mmHg systolic drop indicates impending shock.)
3. If a large amount of fluid is removed, there is a chance that the patient may go into hypovolemic shock.
4. Patient must be on a high protein diet to replace protein lost during dialysis.
5. Connections in the dialysis equipment must be checked frequently to prevent blood loss.

Post-Procedure

1. Make patient comfortable, allowing time to rest.
2. Give patient snack or meal tray if he or she missed a meal.
3. Monitor vital signs as per order.
4. Carry out previous orders.

Your Guide to Urine Collection

Introduction

Your doctor has ordered a special laboratory test for you. This test involves the collection of a urine sample (specimen) for a specific laboratory analysis (test). There are four methods by which this can be done. These methods are a mid-stream voiding specimen, a clean catch specimen, a catheterized specimen, and a 24-hour (timed) specimen. In this information, you will find a discussion of what each of these methods of urine collection is, why they are done, and how they are done. There will also be a discussion of the most frequently asked questions concerning these procedures.

What Is a Mid-Stream Voiding Specimen?

A **mid-stream voiding specimen** is a specimen collected by starting to urinate, stopping, and then collecting the urine specimen when you restart the urine stream.

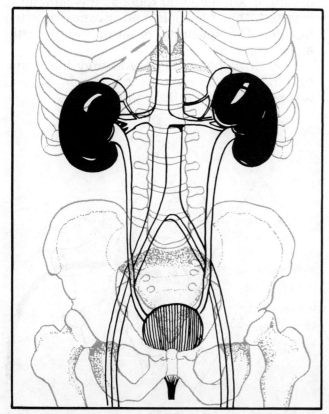

The urinary system.

What Is a Clean-Catch Urine Specimen?

A **clean-catch urine specimen** is collected after you have thoroughly cleaned the skin around the urethral opening. The **urethral opening** is the opening to the canal through which the urine is discharged from the bladder. The **bladder** is a hollow organ that serves as a reservoir for urine.

What Is a Catheterized Urine Specimen?

A **catheterized urine specimen** is collected by the insertion of a sterile (germ-free) **catheter** (small rubber or plastic tube) through the urethra (canal through which urine is discharged from the bladder) to the bladder.

What Is a 24-Hour Urine Specimen?

A **24-hour urine specimen** is a timed collection of *all* urine excreted during that time interval. "All" is a very important word in this definition.

Why Are These Urine Specimens Collected?

Midstream, clean-catch, 24-hour, and catheterized urine samples are collected for diagnostic laboratory analysis.

Is There Any Preparation for These Studies?

No! These can be done on an out-patient basis.

Where Are These Procedures Done?

These procedures are done at home, in your room, a clinic, or a doctor's office.

Who Will Do These Procedures?

All of these procedures are done by you, except for the catheterized urine specimen, which is done by a nurse or physician.

How Are These Tests Done?

1. *Clean-catch—mid-stream specimen*
   These two procedures are usually combined into a single procedure. You will be given

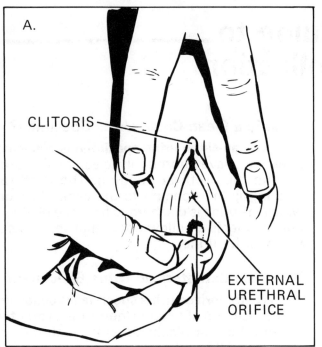

A.

CLITORIS

EXTERNAL
URETHRAL
ORIFICE

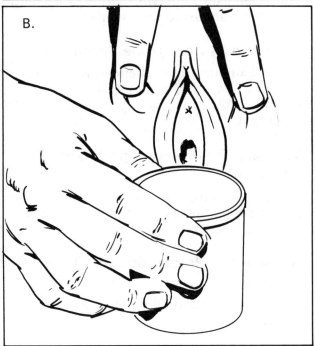

B.

Preparing for midstream clean-catch specimen (female).

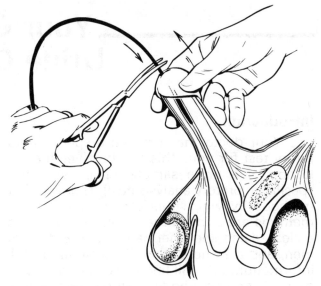

Insertion of catheter in male.

2. *Catheterized urine specimen*

You will be asked to undress from the waist down. You will be assisted onto a table or bed where a pad will be placed under your hips. Your legs will be placed in stirrups or bent at the knees. A sterile (germ-free) field will be established using disposable sterile towels. The skin will be cleaned with an antiseptic (germ-killing) solution. The catheter will be lubricated and inserted into the urethra. If you take a deep breath, it will help you relax as the catheter is inserted. The catheter is then advanced into the bladder. The specimen is taken and the catheter is removed.

After catheterization you may feel some burning upon urination. This is normal, and will be helped by drinking fluids.

a specimen cup for the urine sample, and antiseptic (germ-killing) wipes. When removing the cover, place the flat surface (top) down on the table or shelf. You will be asked to clean the skin around the urethra with the antiseptic wipes. Use each one only once. Always wipe from the front to the back. After this is done, pick up the specimen cup and start a urine stream. Then stop, start the stream, and collect the urine sample in the specimen cup. Be careful not to touch the inside of the cup.

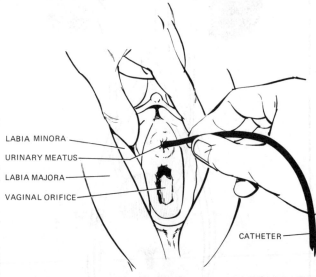

LABIA MINORA

URINARY MEATUS

LABIA MAJORA

VAGINAL ORIFICE

CATHETER

Insertion of catheter in female.

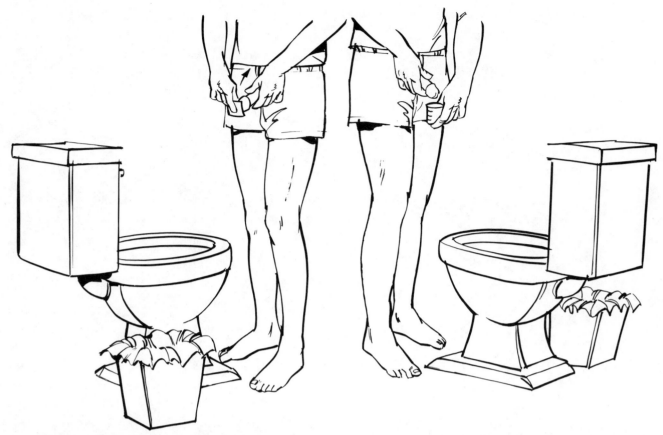

Preparing for midstream clean-catch specimen (male).

3. *24-Hour urine specimen*

A 24-hour specimen is started by throwing away the first urine and then saving all of your urine for the next 24-hour period. There are specific instructions for each 24-hour urine collected. It is imporant to obtain the collection bottle from the hospital laboratory. There may be chemicals in it. Follow the instructions on the bottle. You may be asked to keep the collection bottle on ice. When the 24-hour period is up, the urine specimen will be sent to the laboratory for analysis.

When Will I Know the Results?

When your physician receives the data from the laboratory, you and your family will be told the results of the study.

Will My Insurance Cover These Procedures?

Most insurance companies will cover these procedures. The amount of coverage will vary from one company to another.

Comments and Questions

Your Guide to Urethral Catheterization

Introduction

Your physician has ordered a special test for you. It is called urethral catheterization. In this information, you will find a discussion of some of the most frequently asked questions regarding this procedure.

What Is Urethral Catheterization?

Urethral catheterization is the insertion of a small rubber or plastic tube into the urethra to remove urine from the bladder.

The **urethra** is the pathway from the bladder to the outside opening (meatus) for urine to be excreted from the body.

The **bladder** is the hollow organ that serves as the collection area for urine from the kidneys.

Why Is Urethral Catheterization Done?

Diagnostically, urethral catheterization is done to obtain a sample of urine for laboratory analysis.

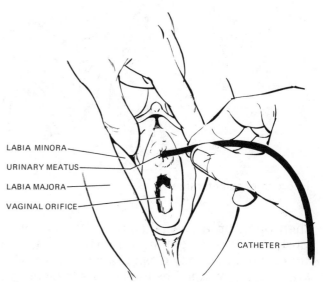

LABIA MINORA
URINARY MEATUS
LABIA MAJORA
VAGINAL ORIFICE
CATHETER

Insertion of catheter (female).

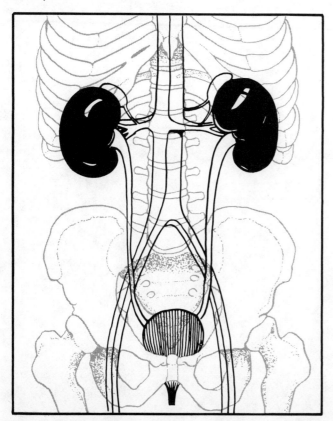

The urinary system.

Therapeutically, urethral catheterization is done to drain the bladder of urine. It may be done at specific intervals, called **intermittent** catheterization, or continuously, called **indwelling** catheterization.

What Is the Difference Between Intermittent and Indwelling Urethral Catheterization?

Intermittent urethral catheterization is done with a straight smooth tube to drain the bladder. Then the tube is removed.

Indwelling urethral catheterization, many times referred to as a foley catheter, is done with a straight, smooth tube with an inflatable balloon at its end. When the tube is inserted and the balloon inflated, the catheter (tube) remains in the bladder to continuously drain the urine. This tube is connected to a drainage bag. It may be left in the bladder for 3 to 5 days.

How Is Urethral Catheterization Done?

The nurse will explain the procedure to you. You will be asked to lie on your back. The drapes will be drawn or the door closed for privacy. A special sheet will be placed under your buttocks to help protect the bed. The female patient will be asked to bend her knees and to spread her legs apart. The nurse will

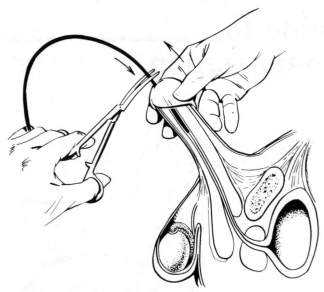

Insertion of catheter (male).

then open up a special sterile catheter set to protect you from getting an infection. At this time, the nurse may clean the pubic area with warm soapy water. The next step is to establish a sterile (germ-free) field by placing sterile towels around the area. (Do *not* touch these towels!) The tube will be inserted. To do this part of the procedure, the nurse will have sterile gloves on to protect the equipment.

Continuing with the procedure, the nurse will open up a special germ-killing solution and wipe off the area where she will put the tube. This again is done to help protect you from an infection.

The catheter (tube) is placed in a special lubricant so that it will move very easily in the urethra. The catheter is now inserted into the urethra. This is not a painful procedure. It will help the nurse if you breathe in and out slowly and relax your muscles. The urine will be drained into a special container and a specimen sent to the laboratory. If the tube is to be removed, this will be done now. However, if it is to be left in, the balloon will be blown up and the tube connected to a collection bag. The tube will then be secured to your leg with tape so you will not pull it loose.

After the procedure, the nurse will help you get cleaned up and make you comfortable. She will allow you time to rest after the procedure.

When Will I Know the Results of the Test?

As soon as the physician receives the report of the laboratory analysis, it will be dis-cussed with you. It may be 2 days if a culture was ordered. A **culture** is a laboratory test to identify germs in certain substances.

Are There Any Complications or Side Effects?

As in any procedure, there is always a small chance for a side effect to occur. However, the diagnostic or therapeutic benefit of having the procedure far outweighs the risk. A few of the side effects that may occur are infection, trauma, or post procedure discomfort. These, however, are rare.

Will My Insurance Pay for This Procedure?

Most health insurance companies will pay for this procedure. The amount of coverage will differ from one company to another.

Comments and Questions

Your Guide to Intravenous Pyelogram (IVP)

Introduction

Your doctor has ordered an examination called an intravenous pyelogram or IVP. This information will discuss many of the questions you have concerning the procedure. For simplicity, we will refer to this procedure as an IVP.

What Is an IVP?

An **IVP** is a series of X-ray pictures of your kidneys (the organs that remove waste and fluid, called urine, from your system), ureters (tubes carrying urine to the bladder), and bladder (organ that holds urine until it is to be excreted or emptied).

Why Is an IVP Done?

An IVP is done to detect any malfunction in one or more parts of the system.

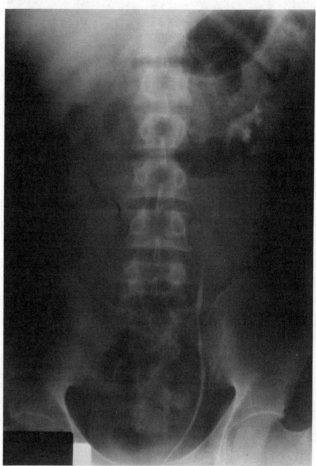

Pyelogram of kidney, ureter, and bladder. (By permission of the Radiology Dept., Lexington County Memorial Hospital, West Columbia, SC.)

Is There Any Prior Preparation?

Yes!

1. If this examination is to be done on an outpatient basis, you will receive a kit and instructions from the X-ray (radiology) department prior to your scheduled appointments.
2. As an in-patient (hospitalized patient), the night prior to the examination you will be given a clear liquid supper (clear soup, tea, juices, etc.). After dinner you will be given a laxative by mouth to help clear the intestine. This enables the radiologist to see the kidneys, ureter, and bladder clearly. The nurse will instruct you later that evening not to drink or eat anything else until your examination is complete. A sign may be

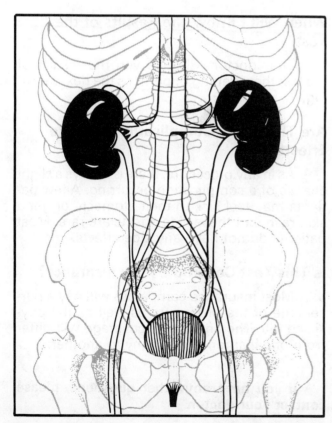

The urinary system.

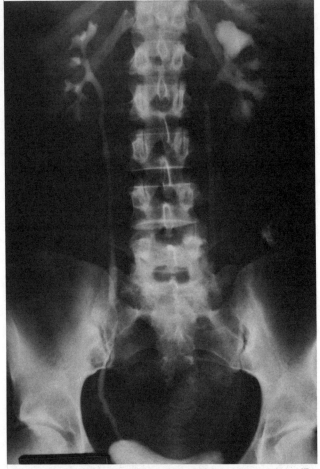

Pyelogram of kidney, ureter, bladder, and urethra. (By permission of the Radiology Dept., Lexington County Hospital, West Columbia, SC.)

placed over the bed or door stating **NPO** or nothing by mouth.

Where Will the Procedure Be Done?

The procedure will usually be done in the radiology department. However, in some hospitals this procedure may be done in the urology clinic.

Who Will Do the Procedure?

This procedure, like many others, is a team effort. The members of the team are an X-ray technologist, a nurse or technician, a radiologist, and/or a urologist. A **radiologist** is a physician who has very specialized training in X-ray procedures. A **urologist** is a physician who specializes in the urinary system.

How Is the Procedure Done?

The morning of the procedure you will be taken to the X-ray department and asked to get into a hospital gown if you are not already in one.

A technologist or team member will ask you if you are *allergic* to anything. This is very important! This test uses an iodine contrast media (dye). It is *very important* that the doctor knows if shellfish or iodine make you sick, or if you have had a prior reaction to the dye.

The team members will place you on an X-ray table and make you as comfortable as possible. A small needle will be put into a vein in your arm. (It is through this needle that the contrast media or dye will be injected.) You may experience a slight stinging sensation and a warm feeling. This is a normal reaction. The contrast media allows for the visualization of the kidneys, ureters, and the bladder.

The X-ray technologist will tell you when he or she is going to take the pictures. It is very important that you do not move during this time.

After the procedure is done, the needle is removed, and you will be returned to your room, or if you are an out-patient, you may return home. It will be important that you drink plenty of fluids the rest of the day to "wash" your system of the dye.

How Long Does the Procedure Take?

The average length of time is about an hour.

When Will I Know the Results of the Test?

Your doctor will give you the results of the test that evening or perhaps the next morning.

Are There Any Complications or Side Effects?

As in any procedure, there is always a slight chance of a complication occurring. A few patients may feel sick to their stomach, or get a skin rash, but these side effects are rare. Most patients do not have any side effects.

Is This Test Covered By My Insurance?

Most insurance companies will pay a percentage of the procedure as well as the physician bill. The amount of coverage will differ from one insurance company to another.

If you have any other questions, please contact your doctor.

Your Guide to Cystoscopy or Panendoscopy

Introduction

Your doctor has ordered a special urologic test for you called a cystoscopy or panendoscopy. In this information, you will find a discussion of the most frequently asked questions concerning this procedure.

What Is a Cystoscopy?

A **cystoscopy** is the procedure of the internal inspection of the bladder and urethra using a cystoscope.

What Is a Cystoscope?

A **cystoscope** is an instrument which allows for the internal inspection of the bladder. It is a lighted, small tube.

Why Is a Cystoscopy Done?

A cystoscopy is done to diagnose bladder tumors or polyps, obtain a sterile urine sample,

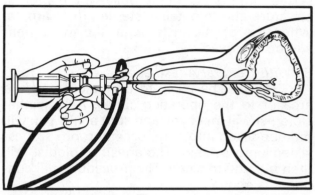
Cystoscope in the bladder.

identify a bladder obstruction due to the prostate, remove foreign bodies, identify urethral structures, obtain biopsies, etc.

Is There Any Special Preparation for This Procedure?

Yes!
1. Food will be withheld until after the procedure.
2. You will be asked to put on a hospital gown.
3. You may be given a sedative to help you relax during the procedure.
4. In some hospitals, this procedure is done under general anesthesia, which would necessitate an intravenous line (small needle put in a vein for fluids and/or medication).
5. This can be done as an outpatient.

Where Is This Procedure Done?

A cystoscopy may be done in a urology clinic, a physician's office, a treatment room, X-ray department, or operating room.

Who Will Do This Procedure?

The cystoscopic procedure is normally done by the team approach. The team is made up of highly trained technologists, nurses, and a urologist. A **urologist** is a physician who specializes in the diagnosis and treatment of the urogenital system.

How Is the Procedure Done?

A. *Without General Anesthesia:*
You will be brought to the cystoscopy room and assisted onto a table. You will be posi-

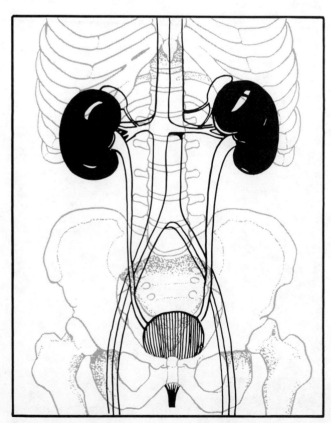
The urinary system.

tioned on your back with your knees flexed (bent) and legs apart. The doctor will then place a numbing medication (anesthetic) into the urethra (canal through which urine is discharged from the bladder) so that you won't feel the cystoscope. Then the cystoscope will be inserted into the bladder to observe the internal structure and to obtain a sterile urine sample. When the physician is done, the instrument will be removed.

B. *With General Anesthesia:*

You will be taken to urologic procedure area or to the operating suites. An anesthesiologist will meet you and start an IV. You will then be taken into a cystoscopy room and assisted onto a table. The anesthesiologist will then put you to sleep. The procedure will continue as above.

After the procedure, if you have had a general anesthetic, you will be taken to the recovery room until you wake up. You will then be returned to your room, or if you are an outpatient, you may return home.

You will be encouraged to drink fluids after the procedure. You may feel a burning sensation after voiding (urinating) or have a small amount of blood in your urine. These are normal side effects of a cystoscopic procedure. Flushing your system with fluids will assist you in correcting these minor problems.

When Will I Know the Results of the Procedure?

The physician will talk to you and your family about the results of the procedure after all of the reports are gathered.

Are There Any Complications or Side Effects to This Procedure?

As in many procedures, there is always a slight chance of a complication occurring. However, the diagnostic or therapeutic benefit of having the procedure done far outweighs the risk. The two most common side effects, mentioned earlier, are burning upon urination and a small amount of blood in the urine.

Will My Insurance Cover This Procedure?

Most insurance companies will cover the procedure as well as the physician's fee. The amount of coverage will differ from one company to another.

Comments and Questions

Your Guide to Urethrography and Cystourethrography

Introduction

Your doctor has ordered a special urologic procedure for you. It is called a urethrography or cystourethrography. In this information, you will find a discussion of the most frequently asked questions concerning the procedure.

What Is a Urethrographic Study?

A **urethrographic study** is a radiography (X-ray study) of the urethra employing an opaque (seen by X-ray) contrast substance or dye.

What Is a Cystourethrogaphic Study?

A **cystourethrographic study** is a radiography of the bladder and urethra, made following the injection of a contrast medium (dye) into the bladder and urethra.

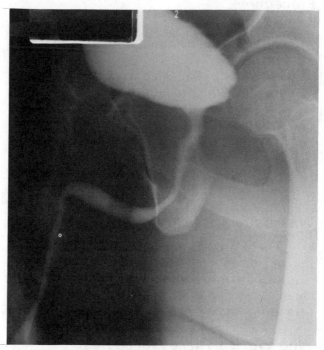

Urethrogram with dye in urethra and bladder. (By permission of the Diagnostic Radiology Clinic, Columbia, SC, Sarah M. Klein, MD, Radiologist.)

Why Is a Urethrographic Study Done?

A urethrographic study is done to visualize abnormalities of the urethra.

Why Is a Cystourethrographic Study Done?

A cystourethrographic study is done to determine the function of the bladder and urethra, as well as the visualization of these parts of the urinary system. If a voiding cystourethrographic study is done, the ureters may be visualized if reflux is present.

What Is Reflux?

Reflux is defined as a return flow. Urinary reflux is urine flowing backward from the bladder to the ureter or urethra to bladder.

What Is the Urethra?

The **urethra** is a canal (tube) through which urine is discharged from the bladder.

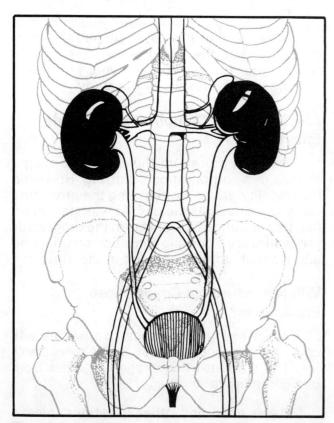

The urinary system.

What Is the Urinary Bladder?

The **urinary bladder** is a hollow organ that serves as a reservoir for urine.

Is There Any Preparation for These Procedures?

Yes!
1. Food may be withheld until the procedure is over.
2. You will be requested to put on a hospital gown for the procedure.
3. These procedures may be done on an out-patient basis.
4. You may be given some medication to help you relax during the procedure.
5. In a few hospitals, a general anesthetic may be given in special circumstances.

Where Are These Procedures Done?

These procedures may be done in a number of places in the hospital or clinic setting. Some of the more common places are urologic clinic, X-ray department, physician's office, and operating area.

Who Will Do These Procedures?

Both of these procedrues are done utilizing the team approach. The team comprises highly trained technologists and two physicians. These physicians are a **radiologist**, who specializes in the use of radiation and radioactive materials for medical diagnosis, and a **urologist**, who specializes in the diagnosis and treatment of abnormalities of the urogenital system in men, and the urinary system in women.

How Are These Procedures Done?

1. *Urethrography*

You will be taken to the X-ray department or to the cystoscopy department. You will be assisted onto an X-ray table and positioned on your back with you knees flexed (bent) and your legs apart. If a general anesthetic is used, it will be administered at this time. Otherwise, a doctor will inject an anesthetic lubricant (numbing medication) into your urethra. This numbing medication is similar to the medication used when the dentist works on your teeth. This is done so you will not feel the insertion of the urethrometer. A **urethrometer** is an instrument used to determine the size of the urethra, and to determine the size of a urethral stricture. Dye will be injected through this tube and several X-ray pictures taken. The urethrometer is then removed.

2. *Cystourethrography*

You will be taken to the X-ray department or to the cystoscopy room. There you will be assisted onto an X-ray table and positioned on your back. Several X-ray films will be made prior to the start of the study. The physician will then inject a dye, via a syringe, into the urethra. There will be a time interval of five minutes post injection of the dye, and then more X-ray films will be done. The physician will then ask you to empty your bladder. (If this is filmed, it is called a voiding cystourethrogram.) Immediately after you have emptied your bladder, more X-ray pictures will be taken. These pictures may tell the physician if reflux is present, as well as to identify any problem areas in the bladder or urethra.

After the procedure, when you return to your home or to your room, you will be encouraged to drink fluids to flush the urinary system of the contrast media. You may have some burning sensation on voiding after the urethrography or have a small amount of blood in your urine. These are common side effects of the urethrographic procedure.

When Will I Know the Results of the Study?

After the films have been studied and other data looked at, the report of the study will be sent to your doctor. You and your family will then be told the results of the study.

Are There Any Complications or Side Effects?

As in any procedure, there is always a slight chance of a complication occurring. However, the benefit derived from having the procedure done far outweighs the risk. As was stated earlier, two common side effects of the urographic procedure are a burning sensation on urinating and a small amount of blood in the urine.

Will My Insurance Cover These Procedures?

Most health insurance companies will cover the procedure as well as the physician's fee. The amount of coverage will differ from one company to another.

If you have any other questions, please contact your doctor.

Your Guide to
Cystography and Retrograde Pyleography

Introduction

Your doctor has ordered a special urological procedure for you. In this information, you will find a discussion of the most frequently asked questions concerning these procedures.

What Is a Urologic Procedure?

A **urologic procedure** is a test that pertains to the urogenital tract in the male and the urinary tract in the female.

What Is a Cystography?

A **cystography** is a radiography (X-ray procedure) of the urinary bladder made after the injection of a contrast media (dye) through a cystoscope.

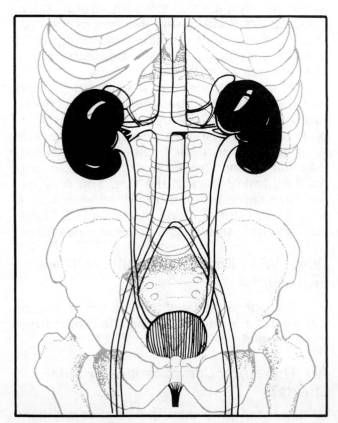

The urinary system.

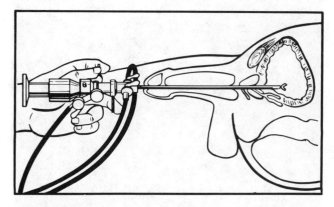

Cystourethroscope inside the penis.

What Is a Cystoscope?

A **cystoscope** is an instrument for the internal inspection of the bladder, ureters, and kidneys.

What Is a Retrograde Pyleography?

A **retrograde pyleography** is an X-ray study of the renal (kidney) collecting system by injection of contrast media into the ureters through catheters inserted with the aid of a cystoscope.

Why Is Cystography Done?

Cystography is done to assess bladder function and to detect the presence of stones in the bladder. This procedure may be done to evaluate the bladder on patients who are allergic to shellfish or iodine. The dye in these procedures does not enter the blood system.

Why Is Retrograde Pyleography Done?

Retrograde pyleography is done to assess ureter and kidney function, and to detect the presence of stones or other obstructions in the urinary system. As in the above, dye in this procedure does not enter the blood system. This is a fairly safe procedure for patients who are allergic to iodine.

Is There Any Preparation for These Procedures?

Yes!
1. The night before the test you will be given a laxative to clean the lower bowel. This

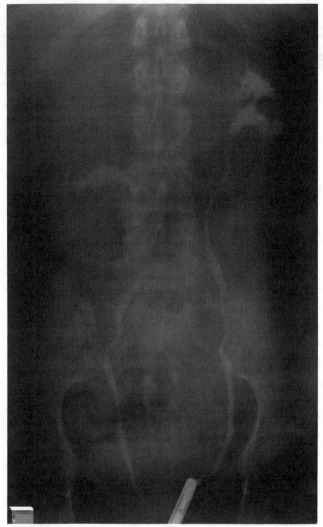

Retrograde pyelogram showing cystoscope. (By permission of the Radiology Dept., Richland Memorial Hospital, Cola, SC.)

Who Will Do These Procedures?

These procedures are done utilizing the team approach. The team comprises highly trained technologists and a urologist. A **urologist** is a physician who specializes in the diagnosis and treatment of the urogenital system.

How Are the Procedures Done?

You will be taken to the cytoscopy room, which is equipped with an X-ray unit. You will be assisted onto a table and positioned on your back with your knees flexed (bent) and your legs apart. If you are going to have a general anesthesia, you will be put to sleep at this time, or a physician will insert some numbing medication into your urethra (canal through which urine is discharged from the bladder), to lubricate and numb this canal so that you won't feel the cytoscope being inserted. The numbing medication is similar to the medication used when a dentist works on your teeth. The cystoscope is inserted into your bladder, and the dye inserted through the cystoscope. If you are having a retrograde pyleography done, very small catheters are inserted through the cystoscope into each ureter and the dye injected through these small catheters. Several X-ray pictures are taken at 15 to 30 minute intervals. The physician will then remove the cystoscope, and will ask you to empty your bladder. If X-rays are done during this part of the procedure, it is called a **voiding cystography**. If general anesthesia is given, this latter study cannot be done at this time.

After the procedure, if you had general anesthesia, you will be taken to the recovery room until you wake up. If you are an outpatient, you may return home, or you will be returned to your room if you are an in-patient. You will be encouraged to drink fluids to help rid the urinary tract of the dye. You may experience some burning on urination or notice a small amount of blood in your urine. These are "normal" side effects of these procedures.

When Will I Know the Results of These Procedures?

Your physician will tell you the results of the procedure after receiving the report from the urologist.

Are There Any Complications or Side Effects?

As in any procedure, there is always a slight chance of a complication occurring. However,

allows the doctor to see the urinary system better.

2. After midnight of the day of the procedure, you will not be allowed to eat or drink anything until the test is over. This is called **NPO** (nothing by mouth).
3. You will be asked to put on a hospital gown the day of the procedure.
4. You may be given a sedative to help you to relax during the procedure.
5. In some hospitals these procedures are done under general anesthesia. If the procedures are done under general anesthesia, an intravenous line (IV) will be started.

Where Will These Procedures Be Done?

The most common place for these procedures to be done is urologic clinic, X-ray, and operating room. The procedures may be done on an out-patient basis.

the diagnostic benefit received from the procedure far outweighs the risk. Two minor side effects that occur, and have been discussed, are burning upon urination and a small amount of blood in the urine.

Will My Insurance Cover This Procedure?

Most insurance companies will cover the procedure as well as the physician fee. The amount of coverage will differ from one company to another.

Comments and Questions

Your Guide to Cystometrography

Introduction

Your doctor has ordered a special urology study for you. It is called a cystometrography examination. In this information, you will find a discussion of the most frequently asked questions concerning this study.

What Is a Cystometrography Study?

A **cystometrography study** is a graphic demonstration of the pressure within the urinary bladder by use of the cystometer. The **urinary bladder** is a hollow organ that serves as a resevoir to hold urine. A **cystometer** is an instrument used to determine pressure in the urinary bladder.

Why Is a Cystometrographic Study Done?

A cystometrographic study is done to evaluate the motor and sensory function of the bladder.

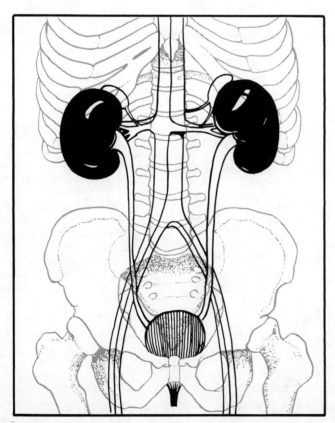

The urinary system.

Is There Any Special Preparation for This Study?

Yes!
1. You will be asked to put on a hospital gown the morning of the study.
2. This study may be done on an out-patient basis.
3. No premedication is needed for this examination. This is a painless procedure.

Where Is the Cystometrography Done?

The cystometrography procedure may be done in several areas of the hospital. Some of these areas are X-ray, urologic clinic, operating area, etc.

Who Will Do the Cystometrographic Study?

This study, like many other studies, is done utilizing the team approach. The team is composed of highly skilled technologists and a urologist. A **urologist** is a physician who specializes in the diagnosis and treatment of diseases of the urogenital tract in men, and urinary tract in women.

How Is This Procedure Done?

You will be taken to the cystoscopy room, where you will be assisted onto a table, and made as comfortable as possible. You will be positioned on your back with your knees bent and your legs apart. This position will facilitate (make easier) the insertion of a tube called a cystometer. The monitor part of the cystometer will allow the physician to measure the pressure within the bladder. To measure the pressure, the physician will insert, via the tube, a given amount of sterile (germ-free) water or salt water into your bladder. You will be asked to tell the physician when you feel the urge to void or urinate (pass your water). The physician may continue to instill the fluid until the urge to urinate becomes involuntary. The fluid will then be removed from your bladder. Your bladder will then be refilled, and you will be asked to tell the physician whether the solution is warm or cold (sensory test). After this infor-

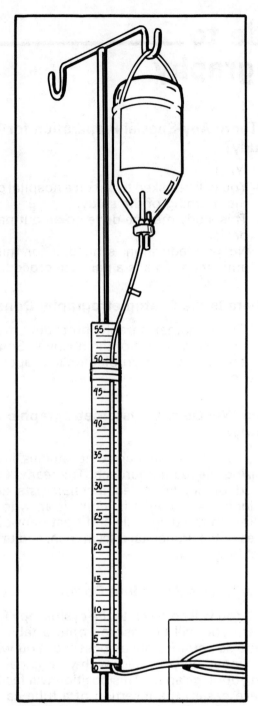

Cystometer.

Will My Insurance Cover This Procedure?

Most health insurance companies will cover the procedure as well as the physician fee. The amount of coverage will differ from one insurance company to another.

Comments and Questions

mation is obtained, the bladder will be emptied, the tube will be withdrawn, and you will be returned to your room. If you are an outpatient, you will be allowed to return home.

When Will I Know the Results from the Test?

Your doctor will tell you the results of the study as soon as the data from the test are received.

Your Guide to
Renal Biopsy and
Percutaneous Aspiration

Introduction

Your doctor has ordered a special test for you. It is called a renal biopsy and percutaneous aspiration. We want you to understand what this procedure is, why it is being done, and how it is done. In this information, you will find a discussion of the most frequently asked questions concerning this procedure.

What Is a Renal Biopsy and Percutaneous Aspiration?

If we define the words of the procedure, we should come up with a suitable explanation: **Renal**—kidney; **biopsy**—excision (cutting) of a small piece of tissue; **percutaneous**—through the skin; **aspiration**—the act of sucking up or sucking in.

Thus the definition for this procedure is: an excision of a small piece of kidney tissue through the skin, using a syringe and needle.

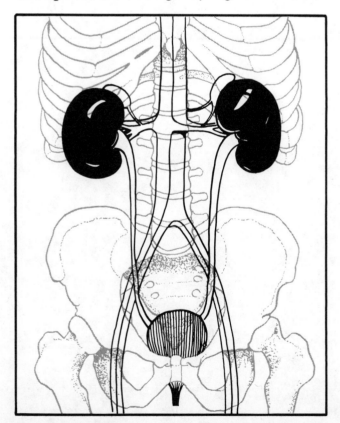

The urinary system.

Why Is a Renal Biopsy Done?

A renal biopsy is done to aid in the diagnosis of acute (rapid start) and chronic (long standing) kidney disease.

Is There Any Preparation for the Procedure?

Yes!
1. You will not be allowed to have anything to eat or drink from midnight (day of procedure) until the test is over. This is called **NPO** (nothing by mouth).
2. You will be asked to put on a hospital gown the day of the procedure.
3. A small needle will be inserted into a vein for use of intravenous fluids and/or medication.
4. Preoperative medication may be given prior to the start of the procedure to help you to relax.

Where Is the Renal Biopsy Done?

This procedure may be done in several locations throughout the hospital. The most common locations are patient's bedside, X-ray, treatment room, or operating room.

Who Will Do the Renal Biopsy?

The renal biopsy will be done utilizing the team approach. The team members will be a nurse, a physician who is specialized in the procedure, and, perhaps, an X-ray technologist and a laboratory technologist.

How Is the Renal Biopsy Done?

You will be taken to the X-ray department or treatment room and assisted onto a table. You will be made as comfortable as possible. A team member will assist you on your side so that the kidney the doctor wishes to biopsy is up. You may be asked to lie on a small pillow. This will assist the physician in obtaining the best position for the renal biopsy.

The doctor will palpate (feel) the kidney. You may feel some pressure from the pushing.

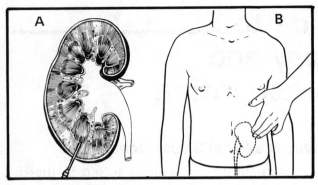

Kidney with needle inserted and location of kidney.

If X-ray (fluoroscopy) is to be used, the doctor may look at the kidney and mark the spot to be entered.

The nurse will ask you to keep your hands at your side, and will then wash the area to be entered with an antiseptic (germ-killing) solution. It may be cold. At this point, the doctor and nurse will place sterile (germ-free) towels around the area to be entered. This is called establishing a sterile field. It is done to help prevent an infection from occurring. Please *do not* touch anything or move now. If you have to change your position, ask the nurse to help you.

The doctor will now inject some numbing medicine into the skin. This may sting, but it will only last a few seconds. This medicine is very similar to what the dentist uses when working on your teeth. When the area is numb, the doctor will insert the needle into the kidney and take the biopsy. You may feel some pressure but should not feel any pain. The needle will be removed and the doctor will hold pressure over the puncture site.

The very small piece of tissue withdrawn will be sent to the laboratory for analysis.

After the procedure, the puncture site will be cleaned with an antiseptic solution and covered with a dry sterile dressing.

When you return to your room, the nurse will check you often and will check your dressing. It is *very* important that you lie quietly for *8* hours and *do not* get out of bed. This does not mean you can get up to use the bathroom. You will have to use the bedpan during this time.

If the puncture area becomes uncomfortable, the nurse will give you something to relieve your discomfort.

When Will I Know the Results of the Test?

Your doctor will talk to you and your family as soon as the laboratory results are received.

Are There Any Complications or Side Effects?

As in any procedure or test, there is a small chance of a side effect or complication occurring. However, the diagnostic benefit received from the procedure far outweighs the risk. A few of the side effects that *rarely* occur are discomfort of the puncture site, infection, and bleeding.

Will My Insurance Pay for This Procedure?

Most health insurance companies will cover the procedure as well as the physician fee. The amount of coverage will differ from one company to another.

Comments and Questions

Your Guide to Peritoneal Dialysis

Introduction

Your doctor has ordered a very special treatment for you called peritoneal dialysis. We want you to understand what the treatment is, why it is being done, and how it is done. In this information, you will find a discussion of the most frequently asked questions concerning this procedure.

What Is Peritoneal Dialysis?

Peritoneal refers to the abdominal cavity where your stomach, liver, spleen, gallbladder, intestines, and other organs are found. The lining of this cavity is known as the **peritoneum** and is used as the semipermeable membrane (filter) for dialysis.

Peritoneal dialysis is a process of cleaning your blood of waste products and poisons. At the same time waste products are being removed, ingredients that are needed by your body may be added.

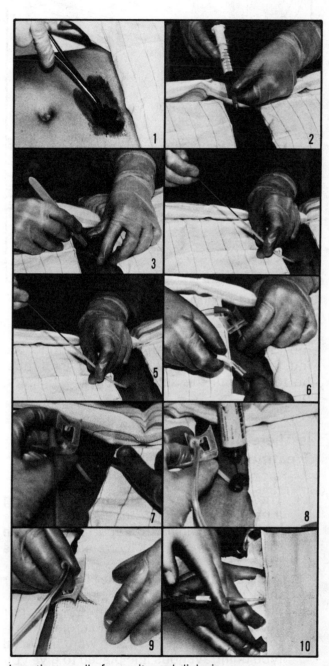

Inserting needle for peritoneal dialysis.

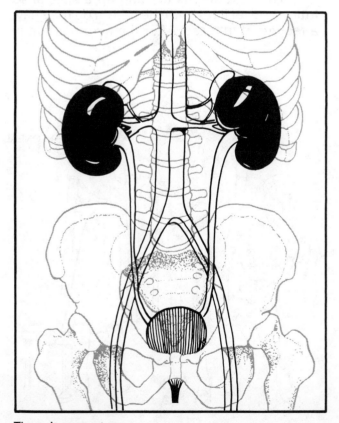

The urinary system.

Why Is Peritoneal Dialysis Done?

Peritoneal dialysis is done to remove poisons and waste products, to remove excess fluid, to help control blood pressure, and to assist in regulating fluid in the body of patients whose kidneys are not fulfilling this need. Healthy kidneys usually do this very special

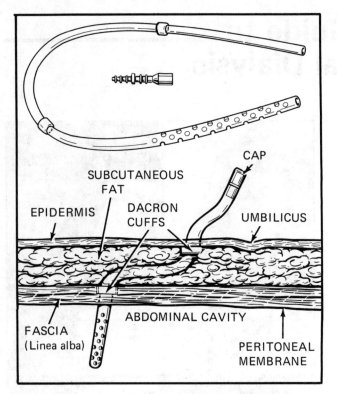

Catheter placement in and through the skin.

EPIDERMIS

SUBCUTANEOUS FAT

DACRON CUFFS

CAP

UMBILICUS

ABDOMINAL CAVITY

FASCIA (Linea alba)

PERITONEAL MEMBRANE

job. However, if the kidneys are not functioning, then a substitute (peritoneal dialysis) must be found until the kidneys begin to function properly.

Is There Any Preparation for This Treatment?

Yes!
1. The physician will talk to you about having a peritoneal catheter (tube) put in.
2. You may be moved to a special unit where the nurses are especially trained to do this test.
3. A few special procedures may be done other than the insertion of the peritoneal catheter. Your doctor may wish to have your heart monitored utilizing a cardiac monitor. The physician may also want a special type of intravenous line placed to give you fluids and measure pressure at the same time. This is called a **central venous pressure line**.
4. You will be asked to put on a hospital gown.
5. You will be asked to empty your bladder.
6. The doctor may give you some medication to help you relax before inserting the peritoneal catheter.
7. Once the catheter is in place, it is used for all of your treatments.

Where Will This Procedure Be Done?

This procedure may be done at the bedside, in a special dialysis unit, or in some cases, at home. (This is called **ambulatory peritoneal dialysis.**)

Who Will Do the Peritoneal Dialysis Treatment?

The peritoneal dialysis treatment is done utilizing the team approach. The team is composed of your doctor, a nephrologist, and nurses. A **nephrologist** is a doctor who specializes in the diagnosis and treatment of kidney disease.

How Is Peritoneal Dialysis Done?

A nurse will explain the procedure to you and make you comfortable. She will take your vital signs (temperature, pulse, and blood pressure) and weigh you. If this is the very first time that you are going to have peritoneal dialysis, your doctor or a surgeon will numb a small area of skin a little lower than your stomach. This may sting but it will only last a few seconds. He will then put a plastic catheter (tube) into this area and sew it in so it will not come out.

The next step is to hang up a special solution and let it run into the tube. You may have a feeling of fullness. After the fluid has run in,

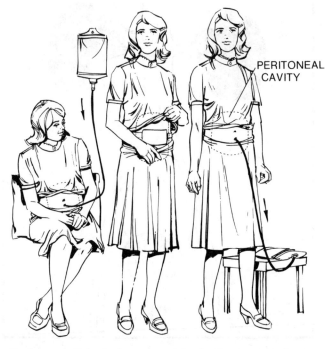

PERITONEAL CAVITY

Peritoneal dialysis done by patient.

the fluid bag or another bag will be connected to the tube and the fluid will be allowed to drain out. The nurse is very busy during this time keeping records, seeing how you feel, taking your vital signs, sending specimens to the laboratory, and making sure that everything remains sterile (germ-free) so that you will not get an infection.

This process is done over and over and may last 48 to 72 hours. During this procedure, you may be allowed to eat if you have a diet. The nurse will turn you from side to side and will frequently care for your skin. She may also ask you to take some deep breaths and cough. All of these things will help you to stay in good health and decrease the chances of your skin breaking down due to inactivity.

After a specified number of exchanges have taken place, the dialysis will be stopped and the tube capped. The area around the tube will be cleaned and covered with a dressing (bandage).

The nurse will be in touch with your doctor for any special orders.

After the procedure, you will be given time to relax. The nurse will again take your vital signs and answer any questions you may have. She will continue to make you as comfortable as possible.

When Will I Know If the Treatments Are Helping Me?

You may feel the results of dialysis almost immediately. Many patients will lose weight, become more alert, and generally feel better.

How Long Do I Have to Take the Treatments?

Dialysis is seldom a temporary treatment for severe renal failure. Your doctor will discuss how you are doing, what type of treatments will be necessary, and how long the treatments will be necessary.

Are There Any Complications or Side Effects?

As in any procedure, there is always a chance of side effects or complications occurring. However, the therapeutic value of the procedure far outweighs the risk. A common side effect is the feeling of fullness during dialysis. Other rare side effects include infection, perforation, low blood pressure, nausea, or fistula (an abnormal connection between two body tissues).

Will My Insurance Cover These Treatments?

Most insurance companies will cover these treatments as well as the physician fees. The amount of coverage will differ from one company to another.

Comments and Questions

Your Guide to
A-V Shunt, Fistula, and Graft Insertion

Introduction

Your physician has ordered a special procedure for you. It is called an arteriovenous shunt, fistula, or graft. In this information, you will find a discussion of the most frequently asked questions concerning the procedure.

What Is an Arteriovenous (A-V) Shunt, Fistula or Graft?

An **A-V shunt** is an alternate pathway or bypass between an artery and vein by surgical means.

An **A-V fistula** is an abnormal (surgically performed) pathway between two surfaces (artery and vein).

A **graft** is a portion of tissue or man-made material used to replace a part of the body. An **A-V graft** is a pathway between an artery and a vein.

Why Is an A-V Shunt, Fistula, or Graft Done?

One of these procedures is done for patients whose kidneys do not function properly (renal failure). It is a pathway by which the blood may be cleaned by an artificial method.

Is There Any Preparation for the Insertion of a Shunt, Fistula or Graft?

Yes!
1. You will not be allowed to eat or drink anything by mouth from midnight before the

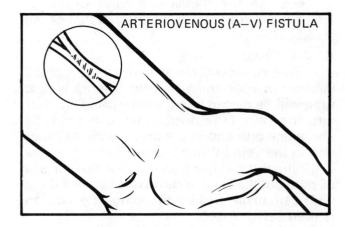

ARTERIOVENOUS (A–V) FISTULA

procedure until after the procedure is done. This is called NPO.
2. You will be asked to put on a hospital gown the day of the procedure.
3. A small needle will be placed into a vein for use of intravenous fluids and/or medication.
4. Preoperative medication may be given prior to the procedure to help you to relax.

Where Is the Procedure Done?

In most hospitals, this procedure will be done in the operating room.

Who Will Do the Procedure?

The shunt, graft, or fistula will be done by a surgeon.

How Are the Procedures Done?

You will be taken to the operating room or a patient waiting room where a small needle

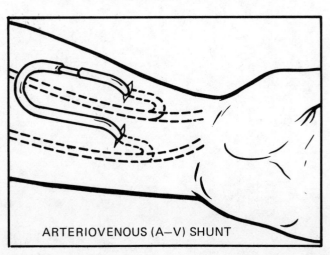

ARTERIOVENOUS (A–V) SHUNT

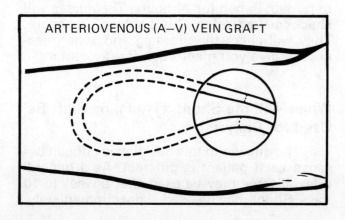

ARTERIOVENOUS (A–V) VEIN GRAFT

will be put in your vein, if you do not already have one.

When it is time to have the procedure done, you will be taken by stretcher to an operating room and assisted onto a table. An anesthetist will then give you some medicine to put you to sleep. An **anesthetist** is a nurse or doctor who specializes in drugs and gases that cause sleep.

A. *A-V Shunt*

Your surgical doctor will make a very small incision in your ankle or wrist. Then a plastic tube will be placed into the artery and another into the vein. (The doctor may use a Y tube and place one end in the artery and the other end in the vein.) When this has been done, he will tunnel the tubes (place under the surface of skin) out the small incision and connect them with a small piece of teflon tubing. The incision is then sewn closed.

B. *A-V Fistula:*

Your surgical doctor will make a very small incision in one of your wrists. After finding an adequate size artery and a vein, the doctor will make a very tiny incision in the side of both of them, and sew the edges of both of the blood vessels together, creating a single opening. This opening is about 4-8mm long. The incision is then sutured closed.

C. *A-V Graft:*

Your surgical doctor will make a small incision in your forearm, wrist or upper arm. The most common place is the forearm. He will then take man-made or animal tissue (the graft) and tunnel it under the skin. At this time, one end is connected into the artery and the other end into the vein. The incision is then sutured closed.

After the procedure, if you had general anesthesia, you will be taken to the recovery room until you wake up. At that time, you will be returned to your room. Your arm or leg will be elevated on a pillow and you may be asked to remain in bed for 24 hours. The nurses will check you very often. This is normal procedure. They will check the dressing and, when necessary, give you medication for discomfort.

When Will the Shunt, Fistula, or Graft Be Used for Dialysis?

The answer to this question is difficult because each patient is different. As a general rule, all three may be used after a week to 10 days. Shunt may be used almost immediately.

Are There Any Complications or Side Effects?

As in any procedure, there is always a small chance of a complication occurring. However, the therapeutic benefit of having it done far outweighs the risk. Some side effects that may occur are bleeding at the site, infection, discomfort at the site and, in very rare circumstances, a blood clot forming.

Will My Insurance Cover This Procedure?

Most insurance companies will cover the procedure as well as the physician fee. The amount of coverage will differ from one company to another.

Comments and Questions

Your Guide to Hemodialysis

Introduction

Your doctor has ordered a very special treatment for you called hemodialysis. We want you to understand what this treatment is, why it is being done, and how it is done. In this information, you will find a discussion of the most frequently asked questions concerning the procedure.

What Is Hemodialysis?

Hemodialysis is a process of cleaning your blood of waste products and poisons. At the same time, ingredients may be added to the blood to help your body.

Why Is Hemodialysis Done?

In the normal person, the kidneys act as filters to remove waste products from the body. However, if your kidneys do not function properly, they cannot perform this important job. Thus, hemodialysis is done to take over the function of the kidneys—removing waste material.

Is There Any Preparation for This Treatment?

Yes!
1. Your physician will talk to you about having a shunt, fistula, or graft inserted prior to the start of dialysis. These are all methods of obtaining blood from veins and arteries.
2. Your physician and dietitian will give you a special diet that *must* be adhered to.
3. You may be asked to put on a hospital gown.
4. You will be taken to a special unit called a dialysis unit. You may go in a wheel chair or in your bed.
5. This procedure may be done on an outpatient basis.

Where Will This Procedure Be Done?

The most common places for hemodialysis are the hemodialysis clinic, a hospital hemodialysis clinic, and it may even be done at the bedside.

Who Will Do the Hemodialysis Procedure?

The hemodialysis procedure is done by the team approach. The team is comprised of highly trained technologists, nurses, and a nephrologist. A **nephrologist** is a physician who specializes in the diagnosis and treatment of kidney disease.

How Is the Hemodialysis Procedure Done?

You will be taken to the dialysis unit where you will be helped onto a dialysis chair (very much like a recliner chair). A nurse or technologist will weigh you and take your vital signs (pulse, temperature, blood pressure). You will be made comfortable as the nurse or technologist starts to connect you to the dialysis machine. This is done by using your shunt, fistula, or graft. You may feel an initial stick of a needle

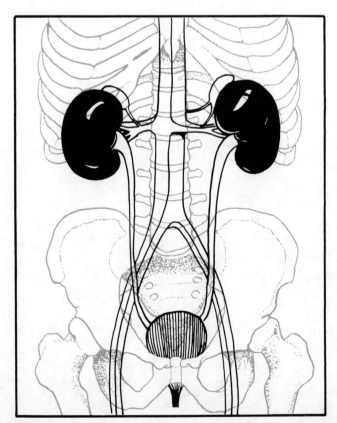

The urinary system.

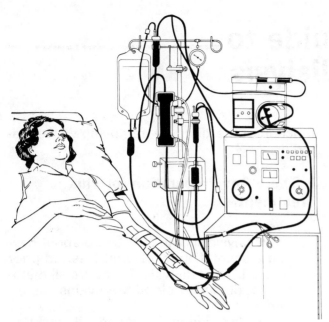
Patient and renal dialysis machine.

but that is all you will feel. Once you are connected to the machine, the nurse or technologist will monitor your vital signs and may send a sample of your blood to the lab for analysis.

During the time you are on the dialysis machine, the nurse or technologist will check the settings, tubing, ask you how you feel, take blood samples, and check your vital signs. Often you will be given lunch while being dialyzed.

The nurse will be in touch with your doctor for any special orders.

At the end of the specified amount of time (which varies from one patient to another), you will be taken off of the machine and returned to your room.

After the procedure, you will be given time to relax and will be given a snack if you missed a meal. The nurse will monitor your vital signs, check the shunt, fistula, or graft, and follow out any new physician orders.

When Will I Know If the Treatments Are Helping Me?

You may feel the results from hemodialysis almost immediately. Many patients will lose weight, and become more energetic and mentally alert after hemodialysis.

How Long Do I Have To Take the Treatments?

Dialysis is seldom a temporary treatment. Your physician will discuss in detail with you what type of treatments, how often it will be needed, and where it will be done.

Are There Any Complications or Side Effects?

There are a few temporary side effects that may occur during the treatment but the nurse or technologist monitors you for these carefully. Some of these may be low blood pressure, feeling faint, or nauseated. Another more serious side effect may be an infection. Extreme care is taken to minimize any chances of side effects.

Will My Insurance Cover These Treatments?

Most insurance companies will cover these treatments as well as the physician fee. The amount of coverage will differ from one company to another.

Comments and Questions

7

Carbohydrate Metabolism Laboratory Procedures

Fasting Blood Sugar (FBS)

The FBS examination is the measurement of the plasma glucose level after a 6 to 12 hour period of fasting.

This procedure is done as a screening test for diabetes mellitus and to monitor drug or dietary therapy in known diabetics.

Nurse's Responsibilities

Pre-Test
1. Explain procedure to patient.
2. Keep the patient NPO post midnight until the procedure has been completed.
3. Withhold diabetic medications or tell laboratory they have been given.
4. Instruct patient not to smoke.

Precautions
1. Observe patient for signs of hypoglycemia (restlessness, nervousness, weakness, diaphoresis, etc.). Notify physician if symptoms are severe.

Post-Procedure
1. Resume previous orders.
2. Order late tray for patient.
3. Check needle site for hematoma.

Glucose Tolerance Test (GTT)

The glucose tolerance examination is the most precise test for the evaluation of borderline cases of diabetes mellitus.

The examination is done to confirm the diagnosis of diabetes mellitus and to aid in the diagnosis of hypoglycemia and other carbohydrate metabolism disorders.

Nurse's Responsibilities

Pre-Test
1. Explain the procedure to the patient.
2. Review the medications that the patient is presently taking to ensure that they will not interfere with the examination.
3. Explain the importance of not eating or drinking anything past midnight.
4. Tell the patient to refrain from smoking before and during the examination.
5. Encourage the patient to drink water to promote urination.

Precautions
1. Many medications can interfere with this examination. List the medications the patient is presently taking. If the patient is on medication that will interfere with the test, notify the doctor and lab.
2. Exercise can change the results of the examination. Instruct the patient to take a book or magazine along and prepare to be quiet for a 3 to 5-hour period.
3. Symptoms of hypoglycemia may occur. Instruct the patient to notify the laboratory personnel or the nurse of any abnormal symptoms. If the hypoglycemia attack is severe, notify physician and discontinue procedure.

Post Procedure
1. Provide patient with a well-balanced meal.
2. Instruct the patient that he or she may resume smoking.
3. Medications withheld prior to the procedure may now be given.
4. Check the puncture sites for signs of hematomas. If they are present, instruct the patient that hot packs to the area will help to alleviate the discomfort.

Your Guide to Fasting Blood Sugar (FBS)

Introduction

Your doctor has ordered a special laboratory test for you, called a fasting blood sugar. This information will discuss why the procedure is done, what the procedure is, and how it is done.

What Is a Fasting Blood Sugar?

If we define each of the words of the test, you will have a good idea what the test is. **Fasting**—without food; **blood sugar**—level of glucose (sugar) in the blood. Thus fasting blood sugar is the level of glucose in the blood without eating for a given period of time.

Why Is a Fasting Blood Sugar Done?

A fasting blood sugar is done to determine how much of the glucose (sugar) that is ingested (taken in) daily is used by the body. There is a delicate balance between blood sugar and insulin. **Insulin** is the hormone that allows sugar to be broken down into a form cells can use for energy.

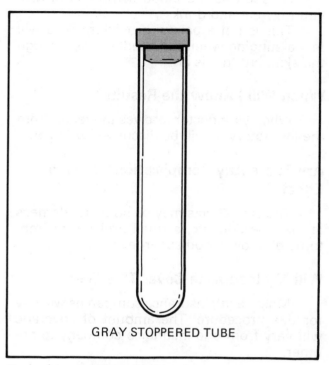

GRAY STOPPERED TUBE

Test tube to be filled with blood sample.

Is There Any Preparation for a Fasting Blood Sugar?

Yes!
1. *Do not eat or drink* anything after midnight of the day the test is to be done.
2. This test may be done on an out-patient basis.

Where Is the Fasting Blood Sugar Done?

If you are a patient in the hospital, the lab person who draws blood will come to your room.

If you are having the test done as an outpatient, the blood will be drawn in the hospital, laboratory, or in a physician's office.

Who Will Do the Fasting Blood Sugar Test?

The blood will be drawn by a laboratory technologist or nurse. It will then be sent to the laboratory for analysis.

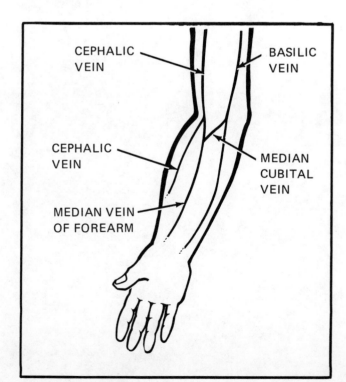

CEPHALIC VEIN

BASILIC VEIN

CEPHALIC VEIN

MEDIAN CUBITAL VEIN

MEDIAN VEIN OF FOREARM

The veins in the arm.

How Is the Test Done?

Someone from the laboratory or a nurse will draw a small amount of blood from a vein in your arm. It will be labeled with your name and sent to the laboratory for analysis.

As soon as the blood sample is drawn, you may eat and drink.

This is not a painful procedure. You will feel a stinging when the needle goes through the skin, but that is all!

When Will I Know the Results?

When your doctor receives the report from the laboratory, it will be discussed with you.

Are There Any Complications or Side Effects?

The side effects may be some tenderness at the insertion site, a small bruise, or symptoms of a low blood sugar level.

Will My Insurance Cover This Test?

Most health insurance companies will pay for this procedure. The amount of coverage will vary from one insurance company to another.

Comments and Questions

Your Guide to
Glucose Tolerance Test (GTT)

Introduction

Your doctor has ordered a special laboratory test for you called a glucose tolerance test. In this information, why the test is being done, what the test is, and how the test is done will be discussed.

What Is a Glucose Tolerance Test?

A **glucose tolerance test** is a laboratory test that measures the amount of glucose (sugar) in the blood at specific time intervals. This is done after you eat or drink a known amount of glucose.

Why Is a Glucose Tolerance Test Done?

A glucose tolerance test is done to determine how well the body utilizes sugar.

Is There Any Preparation for the Procedure?

Yes!
1. The night before the test, do not eat or drink anything after midnight.

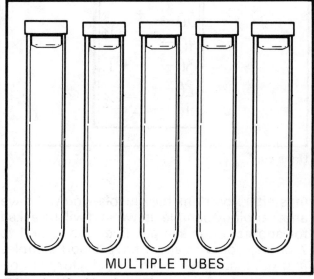

MULTIPLE TUBES

Test tubes for blood samples.

2. This procedure may be done on an outpatient basis.
3. Do not smoke prior to or during the procedure.
4. If taking medication, make sure the doctor and the laboratory know what the medications are.

Where Is the Procedure Done?

If you are in the hospital, your test may be done in your room, or in the lab. If you are an out-patient, report to the hospital or biomedical laboratory.

Who Will Do the Glucose Tolerance Test?

This test will be done by a laboratory technologist. The blood and urine will be sent to the laboratory for analysis.

How Is the Glucose Tolerance Test Done?

Early in the morning a laboratory technologist will draw a small amount of your blood and ask for a urine sample. This is called a **fasting blood sugar**. You will be asked to drink a bottle of **glucola**. It is a very thick and sweet drink. If you smoke, you will be asked to refrain from it until after the test is over. Thirty min-

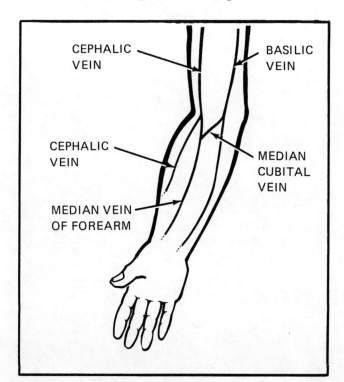

CEPHALIC VEIN

BASILIC VEIN

CEPHALIC VEIN

MEDIAN CUBITAL VEIN

MEDIAN VEIN OF FOREARM

The veins in the arm.

Urine cup.

utes after you drink the glucola, you will have another blood sample drawn and will be asked for another urine sample. Every hour for 1 to 7 hours, you will again have blood samples and urine samples taken. The doctor who ordered the test will decide how many hours it is to run.

After the procedure, you will be allowed to eat, drink, and smoke.

When Will I Know the Results?

The laboratory analysis report will be sent to your physician, who will then talk to you about the results.

Are There Any Complications or Side Effects?

You may experience some discomfort at the puncture sites. Some individuals may experience nausea, perspiring, nervousness, restlessness, and hunger. If these symptoms do occur, tell the laboratory technologist.

Will My Insurance Cover This Procedure?

Most insurance companies will pay for the test. The amount of coverage will vary from one insurance company to another.

Index

Thoracentesis, 61, 75–76
   indications for, 61, 75
   nurse's responsibilities, 61
   procedure, 76
   side effects, 76
Thoracostomy, closed chest tube, 62, 79–80
   indications for, 62, 79
   nurse's responsibilities, 62
   procedure, 79
Thrombus, 54
Thyroid, nuclear study, 2
Tomography, computerized axial. *See* CAT scan

Ultrasonography. *See* Ultrasound
Ultrasound, 1, 5–6
   abdominal picture, 6
   cardiac, 37
   vs nuclear study, 7
   nurse's responsibilities, 1
   obstetric, 5
   real-time, 5
Upper GI and small bowel series, 81, 87–88
   indications for, 81, 87
   nurse's responsibilities, 81
Ureter, pyelogram, 125, 126. *See also* Intravenous pye-
      lography
Urethra, 129
   catheterization. *See* Urethral catheterization
   pyelogram, 126. *See also* Intravenous pyelography
   urethrogram, 129. *See* Cystourethrography, Urethrog-
      raphy
Urethral catheterization, 113
   in female, 123
   in male, 124
   indications for, 113, 123

intermittent vs indwelling, 123
   nurse's responsibilities, 113
   procedure, 124
   side effects, 124
Urethrography, 114, 129–130
   indications for, 114, 129
   nurse's responsibilities, 114–115
   procedure, 130
   side effects, 130
Urinary reflux, 129
Urinary system, 119, 123, 125, 127, 129, 131, 135, 137,
      139, 145
Urine collection, 113, 119–121
   24-hour specimen, 113, 119, 121
   catheterized specimen, 113, 119, 120
      in female, 120
      in male, 120
   clean catch specimen, 113, 119, 120
      in female, 120
      in male, 121
   midstream specimen, 113, 119, 120
      in female, 120
      in male, 120
   nurse's responsibilities, 113
Urologic procedures, 113–146, *See also* specific proce-
      dures

Vectorcardiography, 33, 37, 40
   indications for, 33, 38
   vectorcardiogram, 39
Venograms, 3, 13

X-ray
   vs CAT scan, 2, 11
   chest, 60, 69–70